Case Studies in Communication Sciences and Disorders

Dennis C. Tanner
Northern Arizona University

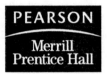
PEARSON

Merrill
Prentice Hall

Upper Saddle River, New Jersey
Columbus, Ohio

Library of Congress Cataloging-in-Publication Data

Tanner, Dennis C.
   Case studies in communication sciences and disorders / Dennis C. Tanner.—1st ed.
     p. cm.
   Includes bibliographical references and index.
   ISBN 0-13-142466-1
   1. Communicative disorders. 2. Communicative disorders—Case studies. I. Title.

RC423.T2638 2006
616.85'5—dc22

2004030125

Vice President and Executive Publisher: Jeffery W. Johnston
Acquisitions Editor: Allyson P. Sharp
Editorial Assistant: Kathleen S. Burk
Production Editor: Sheryl Glicker Langner
Production Coordination: *The GTS Companies*/York, PA Campus
Design Coordinator: Diane C. Lorenzo
Cover Designer: Jason Moore
Cover image: Corbis
Production Manager: Laura Messerly
Director of Marketing: Ann Castel Davis
Marketing Manager: Autumn Purdy
Marketing Coordinator: Tyra Poole

This book was set in Times Roman by *The GTS Companies*/York, PA Campus. It was printed and bound by Courier Stoughton, Inc. The cover was printed by The Lehigh Press, Inc.

The case studies in this book are based on real persons and actual events. The author has made every attempt to protect the privacy of the institutions, clinicians, patients, clients, and their families by changing personal names and altering biographical information. In many cases, locale, gender, and age have also been changed. Readers' assumptions about the identity of the individuals and institutions to which the case studies refer are unwarranted, speculative, and conjectural.

Pearson Education Ltd.
Pearson Education Singapore Pte. Ltd.
Pearson Education Canada, Ltd.
Pearson Education—Japan

Pearson Education Australia Pty. Limited
Pearson Education North Asia Ltd.
Pearson Educación de Mexico, S.A. de C.V.
Pearson Education Malaysia Pte. Ltd.

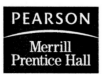

10 9 8 7 6 5 4 3 2
ISBN 0-13-142466-1

This book is dedicated to the men, women, and children chronicled in the case studies, for whom I have the deepest respect. Their forbearance and mettle in facing the adversity of broken communication are tributes to the enduring resolve of the human spirit.

Foreword

Dennis C. Tanner's new textbook, *Case Studies in Communication Sciences and Disorders,* is unique in both concept and implementation. Theories and scientific facts are used as lead-ins to each chapter, and related case studies are presented in a storytelling format. This format is highlighted by clinical sidebars that focus on topic and context, and illuminate questions and issues for the reader. This combination of design features makes the text user-friendly, engaging, and easily readable. The book also covers a wide, traditional range of speech, hearing, language, and communication disorders. This makes it attractive as a companion textbook for introductory courses, for graduate students in clinical practicum, and for practicing clinicians in speech-language pathology, audiology, or special education.

The narrative format of the case studies deviates from the more traditional case study format that often minimizes contexts, details, and event sequences. At first, this format may clash with the readers' expectations of "clinical traditions." However, the story format is in fact inviting, lively, and instructive. Storytelling as a tool for teaching and learning has a long and revered tradition, and Dr. Tanner is adept at using it. It may be worthwhile to take a second look at what a story can provide in building mental models for the learner.

Stories provide the basic structure and often the origin of our mental reference models. They build context-specific personal mental models. In stories, the reader encounters personal experiences and learns how to handle complex situations, deal with dilemmas, avoid conflicts, and observe moral and ethical principles. These details transfer perspectives and visions (Denning, 2000; Wiig, 2004b). If communicated effectively, they can easily be transferred from person to person in story form, and each listener or reader can modify or adapt the contents to create his or her personal models. Even expert clinicians act with reference to the mental models they have stored. Readers will find that they can create their own clinical mental models from the case studies in this book, even though the models may not fit their situation or problem exactly. In other words, readers can adapt the models to fit their own context.

Two kinds of mental models are germane to the case studies that Dr. Tanner presents. The first is an *operational action model,* which provides a practical and detailed approach to a problem or issue and guides us through examples of concrete action steps. The second type is a *specific method model* or *best practices model.* This type of story presents a methodological and often specific approach to dealing with problems and acting to solve them. Some of the case studies in this book provide us with practical models for clinical action. Others present theoretical perspectives and specific approaches for sharing best clinical practices. Most of the case study stories blend the two approaches, and the clinical sidebars with focused explanations clarify both types of mental models for the reader.

Mental reference models are typically internalized and represented in the mind by encoded procedural or cause–effect constructs from stories that have been distilled to extract salient relationships, features, and patterns. Most people, including clinicians, will find it easier to remember complicated relationships and conditions when they are presented, integrated, and structured in the form of stories. As clinicians, we rely on clinical-experience stories to tackle new clinical or educational problems or situations. This textbook is a rich source of good clinical case stories. A quote from a current textbook on how to build and manage personal knowledge in business applies directly to the stories in this book: "*Good stories let us integrate and create coherent and harmonious mental models so that we can understand relationships and make sense of the whole*" (Wiig, 2004a, pp. 110–111).

I hope you enjoy the stories as much as I did. I also hope that you will build new models and review your own internalized models for concepts you may have missed. As I read one of the case studies, I thought of the clinical model I had recently observed and been part of establishing to diagnose and provide intervention for a 4-year old child. I can only state that I and the primary clinician had missed the boat. Through his stories, Dr. Tanner gives us a different perspective to work from, one that has led to better clinical practice. His engaging and diverse case studies can be adapted to fit our own clinical situations and problems.

Elisabeth H. Wiig, PhD

Preface

The reader and writer of the college textbook have a special relationship—the time-honored connection of student and teacher. In this relationship, the writer has the responsibility of providing information in a coherent and orderly way. The writer should prove his or her credibility by citing current and classic studies and the thoughts of past and present authorities on the subject. The writer should present not only his or her own views, but also the basis of these views and their place in the greater scheme of knowledge. The writer is also responsible for introducing material and summarizing it to provide the reader with a context and closure.

The writer also has the responsibility of presenting important and meaningful information in terms easily understood by people from all walks of life while not talking down to them. The words used by the writer should enable and not obstruct communication by capturing and retaining the reader's interest. The writer must continually walk the fine line between overwhelming and boring the reader.

The writer should be tactful when addressing sensitive topics, yet not so much as to be weak or reticent. Thought-provoking ideas are not offensive to most college-level readers, nor should they be. The writer of the college textbook pens in the embrace of academic freedom and has the responsibility to value, protect, and respect that special privilege.

That said, there is no such thing as an unerring writer. There will always be typographic errors, content errors, and faulty sentences; there are no perfect books. It is the writer's responsibility to attempt to achieve perfection in every word, sentence, paragraph, page, and chapter while appreciating the futility of accomplishing it.

The reader of the college textbook has the responsibility of giving the writer the opportunity to live up to his or her responsibilities.

ACKNOWLEDGMENTS

Several people helped me immensely to write this book. First, gratitude is extended to all of the clinicians who evaluated, taught, and treated so many students, clients, and patients and who generously shared their experiences with me. I am also thankful for the help of Rebecca Davis, a talented artist, who provided the illustrations used in this book. Gerald Nadeau, my teaching assistant, did his usual top-notch job in helping me prepare the manuscript. I also appreciate the comments and constructive suggestions provided by the reviewers: Joseph E. Etienne, Western Kentucky University; Virginia G. Walker, Florida State University; Gloriajean L. Wallace, University of Cincinnati; Carla Jones, Washington State University;

Linda C. Badon, University of Louisiana at Lafayette; Patricia B. Schraeder, University of Wisconsin–Madison; Carney Sotto, University of Cincinnati; Teresa K. Graham, Rockhurst University; William R. Culbertson, Northern Arizona University; Kate Battles Skinker, University of Maryland; and Elisabeth H. Wiig, Knowledge Research, Inc.

To the Reader

How vain it is to sit down to write when you have not stood up to live.
Henry David Thoreau

You may be reading *Case Studies in Communication Sciences and Disorders* because your professor required it for an introductory course. Perhaps you are "testing the waters" to see if this discipline is worthy of professional commitment. This book may also be required for an upper-level capstone course or several chapters may have been assigned for a graduate course. You may be in practicum and are reading it to prepare for your first patient. Regardless of your academic and clinical situation, this book is designed to be informative, relevant, and, most important, interesting. The discipline of communication sciences and disorders is exciting, and this book is intended to reflect the awe, wonder, and complexities of human communication, as well as the myriad disorders, deficits, diseases, and disabilities that can lay waste to it.

The chapters in this book address the major communication disorders you are likely to see as clinicians. Each chapter provides an overview of a communication disorder with an emphasis on etiology, diagnosis, and treatment. Although theories are addressed in these sections, the academic reviews are intended to be clinically relevant. These reviews are similar to those found in other books in communication sciences and disorders, but the case studies in each chapter depart from the typical college textbooks you may read.

During the development process for this book, the publisher and I explored several ways of writing the case studies. They could have been written in sterile clinical terminology similar to that of medical and educational reports or in only one style and with little literary variation. However, to make the case studies reflect true clinical practice, we decided to write them in several styles and include detailed patient histories. These histories, including the events leading to the patients' communication disorders, are a fundamental aspect of clinical practice, and they give humanity and depth to the patient–clinician relationship. Clinicians evaluate and treat *people,* not simply their communication disorders, and the case studies provided here reflect that reality.

The cases in this book are based on my 30 years of clinical, academic, and research experience. For confidentiality reasons, and to preserve the privacy of these patients and their families, identifying information has been changed. Literary license has also been taken for descriptive and readability purposes, and some case studies are composites for educational and illustrative reasons. However, all cases reported in this book are based on factual events and real people. I believe this book is both substantive and readable, and provides important and meaningful academic and clinical information. At least those were my goals in writing it.

DCT

About the Author

Dennis C. Tanner received the Doctor of Philosophy degree in Audiology and Speech Sciences from Michigan State University. He is a prolific author of books, diagnostic tests, and treatment programs. Dr. Tanner is the owner of Tanner Rehabilitation Services, Inc., a provider of speech and hearing services in Arizona for 30 years. He is currently Professor of Speech Sciences and Technology at Northern Arizona University and was recently named Outstanding Educator by the Association of Schools of Allied Health Professions.

Discover the Merrill Education Resources for Communication Disorders Website

Technology is a constantly growing and changing aspect of our field that is creating a need for new content and resources. To address this emerging need, Merrill Education has developed an online learning environment for students, teachers, and professors alike to complement our products—the *Merrill Education Resources for Communication Disorders* Website. This content-rich website provides additional resources specific to this book's topic and will help you—professors, classroom teachers, and students—augment your teaching, learning, and professional development.

Our goal with this partnership and initiative is to build on and enhance what our products already offer. For this reason, the content for our user-friendly website is organized by topic and provides teachers, professors, and students with a variety of meaningful resources all in one location. With this website, we bring together the best of what Merrill has to offer: text resources, video clips, web links, tutorials, and a wide variety of information on topics of interest to general and special educators alike.

Rich content, applications, and competencies further enhance the learning process.

The *Merrill Education Resources for Communication Disorders* Website includes:

Resources for the Professor –

- The **Syllabus Manager**™, an online syllabus creation and management tool, enables instructors to create and revise their syllabus with an easy, step-by-step process. Students can access your syllabus and any changes you make during the course of your class from any computer with Internet access. To access this tailored syllabus, students will just need the URL of the website and the password assigned to the syllabus. By clicking on the date, the student can see a list of activities, assignments, and readings due for that particular class.

- In addition to the **Syllabus Manager**™ and its benefits listed above, professors also have access to all of the wonderful resources that students have access to on the site.

Resources for the Student –

- Video clips specific to each topic, with questions to help you evaluate the content and make crucial theory-to-practice connections.
- Thought-provoking critical analysis questions that students can answer and turn in for evaluation or that can serve as basis for class discussions and lectures.
- Access to a wide variety of resources related to classroom strategies and methods, including lesson planning and classroom management.
- Information on all the most current relevant topics related to special and general education, including CEC and Praxis standards, IEPs, portfolios, and professional development.
- Extensive web resources and overviews on each topic addressed on the website.
- A message board with discussion starters where students can respond to class discussion topics, post questions and responses, or ask questions about assignments.
- A search feature to help access specific information quickly.

To take advantage of these and other resources, please visit the *Merrill Education Resources for Communication Disorders* Website at **http://www.prenhall.com/tanner**

Brief Contents

Contents

Chapter Four   Voice and Resonance Disorders   77

Chapter Seven   Dysphagia   151

Chapter Eight   Traumatic Brain Injury   169

Note: Every effort has been made to provide accurate and current Internet information in this book. However, the Internet and information posted on it are constantly changing, so it is inevitable that some of the Internet addresses listed in this textbook will change.

CHAPTER ONE

Language Delay and Disorders

Every utterance is an event, and no two events are precisely alike. The extreme view, therefore, is that no word ever means the same thing twice.

Louis B. Saloman

Chapter Preview: This chapter explores human language and the numerous disorders and deficiencies that can delay or disrupt its development. The definition of language is discussed, and its cognitive, linguistic, and social-communicative aspects are delineated. There is an overview of learning disabilities, and of reading and writing disorders, as well as an examination of language delay and disorders related to attentional deficits, autism, and fetal alcohol syndrome. Case studies are presented of individuals with language delay and idioglossia (twin language), autism, reading and writing problems, mental impairment–mental retardation, and suspected child abuse in a child with language delay.

OVERVIEW OF LANGUAGE DELAY AND DISORDERS

Before the middle of the 20th century, some anthropologists considered **language** to be one of the behaviors separating humans from so-called lower animals. They thought that humans are fundamentally different from the lower species and that the ability to use and understand complex language is an inherently human trait. Although recognizing that lower animals could use and understand *call signals,* anthropologists believed that they were unable to engage in abstract symbolic thought and to generate and understand complex language constructs.

Washoe, a chimpanzee named after a county in Nevada, helped change this erroneous belief. We have long known that chimpanzees do not have the articulatory apparatus to produce complex speech sounds and that teaching them to speak was unlikely given the requisite precise positioning of the articulators. However, several psychologists believed that given chimpanzees' manual dexterity, a modified sign language might be taught to these primates. They began an intensive sign language teaching program, and it soon became apparent that humans are not the only creatures capable of learning and using high level language. Washoe became so proficient with the modified sign language that he clearly was capable of using language that went far beyond a simple call signal system. Since then, many other primates have been taught sign language, and scientists have discovered that other species, such as whales, dolphins, and bees, use language. It is now accepted that humans are not the only species with language. However, humans certainly are more proficient and more capable of mastering this remarkable ability than are other species, and language is one of the likely reasons for our advanced civilization. (For more information on this topic see Chomsky, 1980, and Terrace, Petitto, Sanders, & Bever, 1979.)

Defining Language

There are many definitions of language that vary greatly among professionals. Authorities from a variety of disciplines usually define language as reflecting their professional perspectives. Language is a complex multidimensional aspect of human behavior, and we need a clear definition of it before we can discuss its acquisition, delay, and disorders.

First, language is **symbolic**. Words, whether spoken, written, or gestured, are symbols—arbitrary representations of reality. For example, a person's name is arbitrarily chosen by his or her parents. The letters and sounds of the name create a symbol that refers to the individual. The word is the **symbol**, and that to which it refers is the **referent**. This symbol-referent relationship, or **semantics**, is the core of language and the foundation of linguistic meaning. Whether the symbol is tangible and concrete, such as *comb,* or intangible and abstract, such as *truthfulness,* words are arbitrary symbolic representations of reality.

Second, language is **rule-governed**. There are rules for combining sounds into words and words into sentences, or **grammar**. Specifically, **phonology** is the rule-governed way that speech sounds are sequenced and organized in language. **Syntax** concerns sentence organization, especially word order. All languages are rule-governed and equally able to represent reality; there are no substandard human languages. Knowledge of the rules of language is **competence**, and the ability to use them effectively is **performance**. All normal children are born with the ability to learn language, and a hypothetical part of the mind allowing this acquisition is called the **language acquisition device** (LAD).

Third, humans have several avenues of language expression and understanding. The five primary **modalities** of language are speaking, gesturing, writing, reading, and understanding the words of others. Typically, they are separated into expressive and receptive modalities. The expressive avenues of language are speaking, using expressive gestures, and writing. The receptive modalities are auditory comprehension, understanding what has been gestured, and reading. Performing and understanding simple mathematics are also modes of language expression and reception.

Finally, language is a **social code** that has been agreed on by a particular community. This arbitrary rule-governed system is used by a community of like-minded individuals who accept that system as their mode of communication. Language is a major part of the culture of the people using it.

The following definition of language competence is relevant to communication sciences and disorders and meets the above requirements: Language is the multimodality ability to encode, decode, and manipulate symbols for the purposes of verbal thought and communication. Language per se may also be defined as a symbolic code that is rule-governed, uses several modalities and forms for expression, and serves as a communication code for social and societal interaction (Wiig, 2004). These definitions of language address the multiple possibilities of expression and reception, symbolic encoding, and decoding, and verbal symbolic thought. Each aspect is discussed in this chapter, with case studies demonstrating clinical applications.

Etiology and Diagnosis of Language Delay and Disorders

Many disorders, diseases, defects, and deficiencies can cause language delay and disorders in children. Some are organic and caused by physical irregularities in the child. Others are caused by limited learning opportunities and environmental deprivation. The following are common causes of language delay and disorders in children and considerations in their diagnosis.

Cognitive Prerequisites to Language Development

The role language plays in human thought has been debated for centuries. Some authorities believe that language simply reflects thought, while others are convinced that language and thought are inseparable. Most authorities believe that language facilitates thought and thought facilitates language. Language probably plays a greater role in adult cognition than it does in children because adults engage in more abstract thought.

There are certain **cognitive prerequisites** that are necessary for a child to learn language. These include the sequential development of reflexive behaviors, anticipation, causality, symbolism, categorization, and so forth. A child must develop these abilities, and others, before he or she can acquire and use increasingly higher levels of language. Several tests are available to assess cognitive prerequisites for language acquisition in children, and parents can also be knowledgeable informants regarding stage acquisition (Tanner, Lamb, & Secord, 1997; Tanner, Weems, Nye, & Lamb, 1988).

Mental Impairment–Mental Retardation and Language Acquisition

Certainly not all children with language delay or disorders are mentally impaired–mentally retarded. As is discussed below, there are several language disorders in which children have normal or above-average intelligence. However, mental impairment–mental retardation is associated with delayed or disordered language acquisition. The effects of this condition on language development can be marginal and result in mild language learning deficiencies. Severe mental impairment–mental retardation can profoundly impair or even prohibit functional language acquisition. The American Association on Mental Retardation (2002) provides an up-to-date definition of mental retardation as a disability originating before age 18 and characterized by significant limitations both in intellectual functioning and in adaptive behavior as expressed in conceptual, social, and practical adaptive skills.

Intelligence

Intelligence is a combination of mental abilities that allow the person to think logically, rationally, and effectively and to engage in adaptive problem solving. The operational definition of intelligence is the **intelligence quotient**, a ratio of tested mental development to chronological age (mental age divided by chronological age). Recently, some authorities have expanded the definition of intelligence to include other categories in addition to verbal and performance abilities. Kagan and Kagan (1998) propose eight intelligences, each with adaptive implications: verbal/linguistic (word smart), logical/mathematical (logic/math smart), visual/spatial (art/space smart), musical/rhythmic (music smart), bodily/kinesthetic (body smart), naturalist (nature smart), interpersonal (people smart), and intrapersonal (self smart). "The claim for all of these cognitive styles is that across a wide range of types of information, a person approaches information with a consistent style" (Kagan & Kagan, 1998, p. 3.5).

Several factors must be considered in the diagnosis of mental impairment–mental retardation. This diagnosis requires the individual's intelligence quotient to fall two or more standard deviations below the mean, the condition must occur during the developmental period, and it must impair adaptive behaviors. The most controversial aspect of the diagnosis of mental impairment–mental retardation is intelligence testing.

The intelligence quotient can be compared to other mental test scores, and levels of retardation can be determined. Individuals with mild and moderate mental impairment–mental retardation are sometimes labeled **borderline** and **educable**, respectively, and they either live and work independently or have some experiences in sheltered environments. These individuals usually have the mental capacity to acquire language. Persons with more severe mental impairment–mental retardation, sometimes labeled **trainable** or **severe** and **custodial** or **profound**, are usually unable to acquire language, although individuals in these categories may have some potential to learn it.

Linguistic Development

The **linguistic development** of children has been studied for decades, and today we have a good understanding of the stages that children pass through in becoming linguistically competent. By studying individuals and large groups of children, scientists have learned when specific grammatical, phonological, and syntactic processes are acquired. Beginning with the prelinguistic behavior of undifferentiated crying and ending with the acquisition of high level abilities to use and understand grammatical inflections, norms have been created that determine when children achieve these milestones. Although we refine our linguistic competence and performance throughout our lives, by about the age of 6 or 7 years, the structure and foundation of language have been learned (Tanner et al., 1997). Owens (2001) notes that language development is most remarkable in the first 5 years, when 90% of the syntax, morphology, and phonology are learned.

Early Stages of Linguistic Development

Children acquire the structure and form of language during a period of rapid learning. As noted above, the process begins with undifferentiated crying, in which the child's cries

Table 1.1 Manifestations of Linguistic Disorders

Relatively uniform delay or deficiency in all linguistic functions
Delay or deficiency in one or more linguistic functions, while others are normal
Delayed or deficient linguistic functions, with one or more aspects disproportionately delayed or deficient
Delayed or disordered linguistic functions, with one or more aspects disproportionately accelerated or advanced

are random and little information is expressed. During the first month, crying soon becomes differentiated, and the child's parents can discern different types of cries for different needs. Studies have shown that mothers can understand six or seven different cries in their infants—for example, for pain, hunger, and the desire to be held. Children continue their linguistic development with cooing, babbling, and combining one, two, and three or more words into longer utterances. The child learns to use and understand linguistic constructs such as those for rejection, notice, possession, cessation, disappearance, and so forth. Grammatical, phonological, and syntactic processes are gradually learned and refined, and by school age, basic linguistic competence and performance have been achieved.

Linguistic Disorders

Linguistic disorders can be displayed in four ways. First, some children show a relatively uniform pattern of delay across all aspects of linguistic development. Usually because of global mental impairment–mental retardation, their general cognitive development is arrested and their linguistic abilities reflect the delay. These children have relatively consistent reductions in all aspects of linguistic development. For example, a child with a chronological age of 6 years will use the grammatical, syntactic, and phonological processes of a 3-year-old. Second, some children have a deficiency in a particular aspect of linguistic development, while other aspects are normal. For example, a child may only have problems with self-expression in writing. Third, a child may experience overall delay in linguistic development, but one or more aspects will be disproportionately impaired. Finally, some children have delayed or disordered linguistic development, but one or more aspects will be highly developed and functional, such as seen in savants. Table 1.1 shows the manifestations of linguistic disorders.

Social-Communication Language Development: Pragmatics

Social-communication refers to the way the child uses language to express needs, feelings, desires, ideas, and so forth. It encompasses **pragmatics**, the functional processes that underlie language. Social-communication aspects of language learning include knowing when, where, and why to communicate. This includes appropriate use of verbal turn-taking, requesting information and clarification, and staying on the topic. We see much of social-communication language development in the way children play games.

Playing is an important part of maturation, and children's games can be viewed as their work. When playing games, children learn through trial and error, and there are few penalties for failure. They are free to explore their environment, try different cognitive styles, and discover aspects of their personality. When the games involve other children, the social-communicative functions of language are learned and practiced. Children play cooperatively by directing, questioning, relating, reasoning, narrating, empathizing, and so forth, thus learning and practicing the social-communicative aspects of language.

According to Owens (1995) and Owens, Metz, and Haas (2000), a child with a pragmatic language disorder tends to let the environment prompt interaction; he or she responds reflexively and rarely asks questions. Such a child is likely to use asocial monologues, have a limited range of communication functions, and experience difficulty with stylistic variations and speaker-listener roles. Through individual therapies and group activities involving cooperative play, the child can be taught to use language to express needs, feelings, desires, and ideas and to practice the functional processes that underlie language.

Learning Disabilities

There are several language-based **learning disabilities**, and approximately 7% of all school-age children have difficulty learning and using language (U.S. Department of Education, 1997). "The school-age population with language-learning disabilities is heterogeneous. There are multiple etiologies for their disabilities, and multiple manifestations of their disabilities" (Westby, 1998, p. 338). Learning disabilities are sometimes referred to as the **language disorder syndrome** (Wiig & Secord, 1998).

Dyslexia and **dysgraphia** are reading and writing disabilities, respectively. (**Alexia** and **agraphia** refer to the complete inability to read and write.) In dyslexia, the person has reading comprehension problems due to grapheme (letter) and word perception difficulties. The disorder is associated with poor phonological awareness and listening comprehension (Catts, 1996). Persons with dyslexia have particular difficulty breaking the **phoneme-grapheme code** (Westby, 1998), the ability to pair a letter or letter combinations with a particular speech sound or sounds, either verbally or silently in internal speech. Dyslexia at the perceptual level involves failure to recognize graphemes. The reader has letter reversals and/or does not perceive their shapes in a meaningful way. Typical of this type of dyslexia is confusing *b* with *d* or *p* with *d*. Other letters may have no meaning, and as a general rule, the more similar the shapes of the graphemes, the more likely they are to be misperceived.

Another type of dyslexia involves loss of word meanings. This is typically seen in aphasic patients (who have lost language due to a stroke or some other type of brain injury), but it can also occur because of learning disabilities in children. The person with this type of dyslexia does not recall the meaning of written words or confuses them with others. The condition is sometimes called *word blindness,* but this term is misleading because the reading disorder is not a result of visual impairment. It usually involves semantics and the patient's impaired ability to decode written language at the word level.

Dysgraphia is the inability to express oneself in writing. Although it may include problems with legibility, it is not due to paralysis or paresis of the hand used for writing.

Dysgraphia can involve difficulty copying geometric forms, letters, words, and phrases. Writing to dictation, as in taking lecture notes and composing legible, organized papers, also presents problems that hinder academic performance in students with learning disabilities.

Reading and writing disorders may occur independently of each other, but they often are found together. Thus, treatment usually involves objectives for both dyslexia and dysgraphia. In addition, speech-language pathologists incorporate **literacy training** into all therapies, particularly those involved with reading and writing.

Literacy Training and Language Disorder Syndrome

Recently, speech-language pathologists have made a more concerted effort to incorporate their clients' reading and writing educational goals into therapy objectives. (For more on literacy and language, see Stone, Silliman, Ehren, & Apel, 2004.) Today these clinicians assume a primary role in children's literacy development. This is reasonable given their extensive knowledge and training in language development and disorders. These therapists bring knowledge and skills to the classroom that enhance children's literacy learning, and they are valuable educational resources.

Hearing Loss, Attentional Interactions, and Attention Deficits

Hearing is sometimes called the *second sense* after the primary sense of vision. However, normal hearing and higher level auditory processing are primary in learning language. They are essential to learning and appropriately using language symbols for speech, writing, and reading. Consequently, a client's hearing must be screened and, if warranted, thoroughly evaluated before diagnosing language delay or disorders. In addition, though children may have normal hearing, their processing of auditory stimuli may be compromised by **attention deficits**. Westby (1998) defines **attentional interactions** as the child's capacity to attend to and discriminate among stimuli. She notes that the behaviors the infant uses to respond to and maintain stimulus inputs can be manifested in several ways, such as visual tracking, smiling in response to a familiar person, laughing, and orienting toward sound. Problems with sound orientation in the infant may be one of the first indications of an **auditory processing disorder** (APD). According to Martin and Clark (2003, p. 209), "Auditory processing disorders is [the term] often applied to children whose recognition or use of language is not age-appropriate and/or is inconsistent with their level of intelligence. Many of these children also have additional learning disabilities that prevent them from progressing normally in their education." More boys than girls have auditory processing disorders, which affect the acquisition and use of language. English (2002) lists early signs of APD, including inconsistent responses to auditory stimuli, short attention span, distraction, frequent requests for repetition of information, and problems with short- and long-term memory.

Auditory processing disorders include **attention deficit disorder** (ADD), and the two diagnostic labels are used by some professionals interchangeably. ADD and **attention deficit hyperactivity disorder** (ADHD) are overused terms and frequently misdiagnosed attention interaction disorders (see Barkley, 1997). The medical management of these conditions and the use of psychotropic medication are also excessive and often inappropriate. Not all unruly children have ADHD. The disorder primarily affects boys, who have difficulty regulating their actions and appreciating the consequences of their behavior. They tend to be impulsive and incapable of inhibiting their statements and actions. These children have deficiencies in mental executive functioning similar to those of some traumatically brain-injured persons, although to a lesser extent. Children with ADD or ADHD display problems in planning, regulating, and monitoring behavior. Thus, pragmatic language development is a primary therapy goal.

Autism

According to Hirsch (1998), **pervasive developmental disorders** occur in about 15 per 10,000 live births and are four times more common in boys than in girls. They include a broad spectrum of developmental disorders that can affect cognitive, emotional, and social development. Language development is compromised in many children with pervasive developmental disorders.

Autism, a pervasive developmental disorder, comes from the Greek word *autos*, meaning *self*, and is the tendency toward morbid self-absorption at the expense of regulation by outward reality (Dirckx, 2001). "The social disfunction [sic] observed in autistic children is never observed in normal children of any age and cannot be accounted for on the basis of mental retardation alone" (Wesby, 1998, p. 188). The etiology of autism is unknown, but is probably neurological and not related to negative parent–child interaction. In the past, some authorities on autism believed it was caused by early poor mother–child bonding, but this theory has since been rejected. Vitamin and mineral deficiencies, infections, diseases, and other prenatal irregularities may cause areas of the fetus's brain to develop abnormally.

Although autism may cause deficits in all aspects of language development, the social-communicative functions are particularly impaired, especially those pertaining to emotional expression and reception. Persons with autism typically do not use speech to interact with others; communication is often limited to a call system and random noncommunicative utterances. Besides exhibiting deficits in pragmatic use of language, these persons typically engage in **perseveration**, the tendency to engage in an act longer than is warranted by the intensity of the stimuli causing it. Related to the perseveration seen in autism is **echolalia**, the repetition of recently spoken words. **Self-stimulation** is also common in autism. It can take the form of oral clicking, hand tapping, eye-strobing (moving the fingers rapidly in front of the eyes to create a strobe effect), and self-abusive behaviors such as pinching and clawing the body. Sometimes persons with autism repetitively strike themselves. The typical individual with autism is mentally impaired–mentally retarded, emotionally detached from loved ones, socially isolated by choice, perseverative, echolalic, self-stimulative, and profoundly delayed in speech and language development. Some persons with autism are **savants**. Although mentally impaired–mentally retarded, autistic savants are highly developed and proficient in a particular musical, mathematical, or psycholinguistic function. **Aspergers syndrome** is an autistism-like pervasive developmental disorder marked primarily by social interaction deficits (Ozonoff, Dawson, & McPartland, 2002).

Fetal Alcohol Syndrome

Fetal alcohol syndrome (FAS) and a milder form of this disorder, **fetal alcohol effect** (FAE), are common birth defects (Tharpe, 2004). FAS is a cluster of fetal defects including orofacial anomalies, spine and limb malformations, mental impairment–mental retardation, language delay, and other disorders caused by ingestion of alcohol by the mother during pregnancy. The severity of the malformations in the fetus appears to be related to how much alcohol the mother has consumed and for how long. Current research suggest that there is no safe level of alcohol consumption for expectant mothers. Children with FAS and FAE have communication deficits ranging from mild pragmatic and social-communication impairments to profound language delay.

Delayed Language Development

Toddlers with delayed language development are sometimes called **late talkers**. "In the research literature, late talkers are typically defined as young children (between approximately 16 and 30 months) whose language skills fall below [those of] 90 percent of their age peers" (Plant & Beeson, 2004, p. 177). Plant and Beeson's review of current research on late talkers suggests that these children tend to be at risk for continued language problems, and that the earlier the diagnosis is made, the better the outcome; young children fare better than older ones. In addition, many children identified as late talkers tend to remain behind their peers in language development. Plant and Beeson conclude that there is no consensus on the types of early language deficits (e.g., poor comprehension, initial severity of the deficits, limited use of gestures and vocabulary) that predicts whether late talkers will catch up to their peers. Clinical prudence suggests that early detection, monitoring, treatment, and follow-up of late talkers will likely prevent language-based educational, psychological, and social complications later in their lives.

Treating Language Disorders and the Individuals with Disabilities Education Act

In 1975, Congress enacted Public Law 94-142, which guarantees students with disabilities appropriate special education services. In 1997, President Bill Clinton signed the **Individuals with Disabilities Education Act** (IDEA) into law. These laws and other federal, state, and local regulations dictate the nature and extent of special education services provided to persons with disabilities. They are particularly relevant to the diagnosis and treatment of language delay and disorders.

All eligible children with special needs are entitled to **free and appropriate** public education in the **least restrictive environment**. To prevent the use of culturally discriminatory tests, language testing must accommodate English as a second language. The tests should be given in the language spoken in the home or administered with the aid of an interpreter. The **Individualized Education Plan** (IEP), sometimes called the **Individualized Education Program**, specifies when the services begin, their anticipated duration, short- and long-term goals, and the criteria used to determine when and whether the objectives have been met.

The IEP also details the extent to which the child can participate in classroom activities. IEP meetings are held annually, and the child's parents or guardians are present. Sometimes the student is also invited to attend. During the meetings, the IEP is reviewed and changes are made in writing to address progress and deficiencies. All parties are required to sign it, although there are provisions for absentees. There are established procedures to protect the parents' and child's rights.

It should be noted that over a 10-year period, issues related to IDEA were the most frequent sources of litigation involving speech-language pathologists and audiologists (Tanner, 2003b; Tanner & Guzzino, 2002).

Children with language delay and disorders require special consideration due to the inherently cultural nature of language. Culture and language are fundamentally related. Language carries a culture's history, customs, beliefs, and values from one generation to the next. It provides an avenue of cultural expression. Thinking in one language is not identical to thinking about the same subject in another language, and some have criticized the verbal sections of intelligence tests as not providing objective, culturally sensitive scores. Speech-language pathologists, whether addressing dyslexia, attentional deficits, autism, dysgraphia, or other language-based disorders, must consider the child's culture when testing, determining goals and objectives, and implementing treatments. Language differences are not necessarily language disorders, and appreciating the relationship between culture and language ensures that language delay and disorders are correctly identified and treated.

Case Studies in Language Delay and Disorders

Case Study 1.1 Language Delay Secondary to Environmental Deprivation

BLAKE

The diagnostic team pulls into town, unloads test after test from the trunks of the cars, and sets up several evaluation stations in the large Head Start center. Today they will screen and, when indicated, further evaluate twenty-three 4- and 5-year-old children. This center is the final stop on the diagnostic circuit; during the past 2 weeks, the team has visited 14 centers and tested nearly 250 children. The diagnostic team has the screening routine down precisely. Earlier in the week, a questionnaire was sent to all teachers who identified children they considered at risk for communication disorders. Although all children will be screened, those whom the teachers thought may be developing communication disorders will receive special attention.

Clinical Sidebar 1.1
Research and clinical practice show that when Head Start teachers are trained to identify children with communication disorders, they are accurate diagnosticians. They are most accurate in referring children with articulation and phonology disorders, but they tend to be overly concerned about early-onset stuttering. It is important that teachers interact with children for at least 1 month to become familiar with their communication abilities before giving their impressions. Do you think that simply asking a teacher whether a pupil has a communication disorder is an adequate screening process?

The purpose of the screening is to detect children who are having problems with communication or are likely to develop them. A series of quick but accurate screening tests are administered as each child passes through the evaluation stations. One clinician interviews the child's parents, if available, and escorts each child from station to station. Most of the screeners are functionally multilingual, and if the home language of the child is not spoken by the tester, the Head Start center has arranged for a parent, teacher, or teacher's aide to be present who speaks this language. Although each station has a particular objective, the testers are encouraged to note any type of communication irregularity they observe.

The first station is for hearing screening. The Head Teacher's office is used to set up the portable audiometer, and it is biologically calibrated. In biological calibration, the clinician screens his or her hearing and adjusts the base loudness levels for the ambient noise. Of course, screening hearing with excessive ambient noise is less than desirable, but it is sometimes necessary. At this station, each child is screened at several pure tone frequencies; if he or she fails two or more of the frequencies tested, then retesting is scheduled. The diagnostic team also has an impedance screening device capable of detecting middle ear dysfunction.

The second station is for voice, articulation, phonology, and fluency screening. There are words to repeat, objects to name, and pictures to describe. The activities have been carefully selected so that each child produces all of the consonants and vowels and talks enough so that fluency can be assessed. The child's intelligibility is tested, and a percentage score is assigned reflecting his or her ability to be understood. This is an important test; unintelligibility can negatively affect a child socially and educationally. There is also a section in the screening protocol for voice quality and loudness.

The third station is for language screening. These tests determine whether the child has age-appropriate expressive and receptive language. They are by far the most time-consuming because there are many aspects to test and lengthy responses are required. At this station, the child names and describes the functions of objects, identifies colors, makes grammatical constructions, and follows commands; the clinician assesses the average number and length of utterances. The teachers' reports are reviewed to learn their impressions of the child's use of language at snack times, during classroom activities, and at play.

At the final station, all of the information is reviewed, and the clinicians, teachers, aides, and parents are questioned about unusual scores and irregularities. Children with below-average scores are given a follow-up screening test to confirm or reject the results. A child who fails the screening is referred for a comprehensive hearing, speech, and/or language evaluation. Because the clinicians recognize that accurate screening of hearing, speech, voice, fluency, and language in children enrolled in Head Start is challenging, they have agreed that if an error is to be made, a false positive is preferable to a false negative. Although they try to avoid mistakes, they are careful in making recommendations for further testing. They would rather refer a child for an evaluation unnecessarily than miss a child with a developing communication disorder.

During the screening, Blake, a 5-year-old boy, comes to the final station. He is described as significantly delayed in learning expressive and receptive language. He speaks primarily in one-word utterances, rarely combines words correctly into two- and three-word utterances, and shows poor grammatical development, phonological delay, and a restricted receptive vocabulary. The teacher's report also shows that Blake is talking at a 2-year level. According to the teacher, Blake lives on a farm many miles from town, is an only child, and, until enrollment in Head Start, had very little interaction with other children. A comprehensive speech and language evaluation is recommended.

The evaluation at the university's Speech and Hearing Clinic confirms Blake's language delay. Tests show that he uses receptive language at a 2-year, 3-month level, and his expressive language is even more delayed. The percentile rank, a test score comparing him to his peers, shows him to be functioning at the 5th percentile, meaning that about 95% of children his age use language more efficiently. Intelligence testing conducted by a neuropsychologist does not suggest mental impairment–mental retardation. The diagnostic team believes the cause of the language delay to be environmental deprivation.

Actually, for Blake, this diagnosis is misleading; he is far from deprived of environmental stimulation. Farm life is healthy, exciting, and exhilarating. Blake has 40 acres of rolling hills to roam, barns and outbuildings to explore, fresh air, and open spaces in which to play. He has his own pony, pet goats, rabbits, and his faithful dog, who accompanies him everywhere. There are daily chores for the young boy, including gathering eggs and feeding the chickens. He rides with his father on the tractor and helps his mother in the family garden. But unfortunately, this rich environment lacks social interaction. Blake has no siblings and no other playmates of his age. He has no one with whom to talk, argue, squabble, discuss, banter, and joke. Consequently, he has not learned the vocabulary of children his age or how to use language pragmatically.

Head Start provides language stimulation, and Blake's enrollment in the program is helpful. However, because of his delayed language acquisition, he sees the speech-language pathologist to learn age-appropriate vocabulary and to develop other aspects of language. The therapy and the Head Start program soon provide the stimulation and conditions necessary for Blake to catch up to his peers. By the time Blake enters first grade, his language is age-appropriate and he enjoys the best of both worlds.

Case Study 1.2   Idioglossia

CHRIS AND KARL

Chris and Karl were not twins, but they were very close in age. Chris was older by 11 months, and when Karl was born, it was too much for their mother. Eventually she took a job in California, leaving the children in the very competent hands of their grandmother. A traditional Navajo, the grandmother lived in a remote region of the reservation, tending sheep, growing corn, and having little contact with others. For nearly 4 years, Chris and Karl played almost exclusively with each other. Their grand-mother spoke little English and was quiet and reserved, rarely talking to the children. Chris and Karl soon developed their own unique language. It was a curious mix of English and Navajo, with several sounds not heard in any language of the Southwest. When Chris and Karl were about 5, their mother assumed custody of them, moved to a small town in New Mexico, and enrolled them in Head Start.

As often happens during screenings, there was little detailed background information about the children. During the morning session, a clinician told the supervisor that she was perplexed about Chris and Karl's language, which appeared to be unlike any spoken at the center. The Navajo interpreter listened carefully to them talk and said that although she could recognize some Navajo sounds, their language was no dialect of Navajo she had ever heard. The Spanish interpreter made similar comments. The Apache bus driver for the center also said that the children were not speaking his language.

The teachers, aides, and diagnostic team watched Chris and Karl interact verbally. What they saw was remarkable and left an indelible impression on them. The boys played together in the corner of the Head Start classroom, ignoring other children and adults. The activity was a block-building game in which the goal was to create a tower. Chris took the lead, pointed to several colorful plastic blocks, and then uttered what appeared to be a four- or five-word statement to Chris. None of the words he used was English, Navajo, Spanish, Apache, or apparently any other established language. But it was functional for the boys, and Karl immediately took the smaller blocks from the tower and replaced them with larger ones. He replied using their unique language, which was understood only by Chris. The adults watched them talk for nearly an hour and were mystified. Their language appeared to have more than 100 words spoken and understood only by the children. Although the language was difficult to assess, it appeared to have a complex grammar and syntax. Interestingly, the boys avoided other children and made no attempt to talk with them in English or Navajo. They refused to allow other children to play with them and physically removed them from the games. The teachers at the Head Start center said that the children were inseparable and would cry when apart.

It would have been eye-opening to study Chris and Karl's idioglossia. Their language could have been analyzed for form and content and a dictionary constructed. What the diagnostic team witnessed was the birth of a new language, and to have followed its development throughout the children's lives would have been enlightening—especially if Chris and Karl had returned to the reservation and continued to mature in relative isolation. But

Clinical Sidebar 1.2

There is an optimal time for humans to acquire language. From birth to approximately the teenage years, children are able to learn language or multiple languages most efficiently. During this "window of opportunity," children do not need formal training; they simply acquire the language or languages to which they are consistently exposed. Although adults also can learn multiple languages at any age, the most efficient time is up to the teenage years. Why do you think it is easier for children than for adults to learn a second language?

of course, the educational, social, and psychological needs of the brothers far out-weighed the scientific benefits of such a study. Consequently, a strategy for eliminating the idioglossia was developed after conferences with the Head Start director and teachers, the boys' mother and grandmother, the social worker, and representatives from the Department of Child Welfare.

Chris and Karl were gradually separated from each other. Initially, they were placed in separate study and play groups in the classroom. Later, Chris was placed in the morning session and Karl in the afternoon session. At first, this separation was distressing. They cried for each other and refused to interact with the other children. Because they were in different sessions, they also had less interaction with each other after preschool. Chris and Karl were also placed in language therapy. They were seen daily by a certified speech-language pathologist.

The language therapy was unique in several ways. One of the main differences between traditional language therapy and that given to Chris and Karl was that their vocabulary needed to be unlearned. The symbols they had used to refer to thoughts, feelings, and objects were unique to them, but were not meaningful to others and therefore had to be eliminated. For example, while naming activities using flash cards, the clinician would correct Chris or Karl when they called a knife a *nuga,* saying, "No, it is not a 'nuga,' it is a 'k–n–i–f–e.'" In addition, the clinician did not grant their requests or talk to them when they spoke in their unique language even if what they were saying was understood.

Another unique aspect of the boys' language therapy involved the role of idioglossia in thought. Although much of their language simply reflected their thought processes, they also were beginning to process information internally with inappropriate symbols. This was particularly apparent during categorization activities. For example, they had to relearn shapes and colors by categories and redefine their perceptual boundaries.

Much of the language therapy provided to Chris and Karl was atypical because of the idioglossia, and the social-communicative (pragmatic) aspects of language required special goals and methods of achieving them. Both boys had short conversations with their schoolmates, but their communications were often ineffectual. They seemed not to understand the idea of taking turns and never initiated a conversation.

Although Navajo cultural norms concerning social communication were respected, goals and therapies were established to improve Chris and Karl's pragmatic language skills. They first were seen individually, and the clinician worked to increase the length of conversational episodes and improve their effectiveness. The boys were shown how turn-taking works and when to initiate a conversation. Then, in small groups with other children who had similar problems, they practiced the social-communicative functions of language under the clinician's direction.

Chris and Karl received therapy throughout the Head Start program and the elementary grades. Gradually, their language abilities improved to age-specific levels. However, their mother reported that the boys had a special bond, and when they were alone, they frequently used the unique language they had developed while growing up on the reservation. The idioglossia was a testimony to that special bond.

Case Study **1.3**   Autism in a Residential Treatment Facility

MIKEY

Clarene knew that most people simply did not understand how an autistic child dramatically alters family life. The birth of any child has a strong effect on the family's relationships, routines, and finances, but the special needs of a child with autism can turn a household upside-down. Clarene and her husband, Steven, met the challenges of autism head on, and Mikey's Moonshadow Ranch is the result. The ranch has taken 20 years to create, but it now provides eight autistic adults, six men and two women, an exemplary residential treatment facility.

At first, Michael, or "Mikey," as everyone called him, appeared normal and acted like most infants. However, there were early signs that Mikey's development was atypical. The first sign was the lack of bonding. Mikey was aloof and distant. He was *tactile defensive*, not seeking or appearing to enjoy physical intimacy. He tended to treat his parents as objects, showing little interest in them and even less affection. Another early sign of autism was self-stimulation. Mikey used several forms, but especially putting his spread-out fingers close to his eyes and rapidly moving them up and down, creating a strobe effect. This is his favorite "stimming" behavior, and he frequently uses it when anxious or distressed.

Mikey's Moonshadow Ranch is set on 10 acres of rolling hills. A small creek runs through the center of the ranch, and several weeping willow and oak trees border it. The ranch is fenced with wire and steel t-posts, and the corrals are made of wooden panels carefully painted by the "ranchers." There is an old red barn with a hay loft and several outbuildings. In the center of the ranch are the bunkhouse, main home, mess hall, and swimming pool.

Clinical Sidebar 1.3
Prolonged and excessive use of medication can cause tardive dyskinesia, characterized by muscular jerks, tremors, and writhing-twisting movements. When tardive dyskinesia affects speech muscles, unwanted and abnormal sounds can be produced while speaking. What other behaviors can be caused by prolonged and excessive use of medications?

There are no typical days at Mikey's Moonshadow Ranch, but they usually start early in the morning when one of the ranchers disrupts the quiet of the bunkhouse. The aide who sleeps in the bunkhouse awakens the rest of the male ranchers in time for breakfast. (The two women sleep in the main house with Clarene, Steven, and another aide.) Most of the men can dress themselves if their clothes have been laid out the night before. They then go to the mess hall for breakfast, although some wander and need coaxing and direction. Mikey is usually first at the table and has the biggest appetite. The two aides help the ranchers with the meal and try to keep spilled liquid and food to a minimum. This morning the orange juice is more tart than usual, causing Mikey to say repeatedly, "Dentist," perhaps referring to the taste of the juice in his mouth or, as often happens, apparently referring to nothing at all. He also begins "strobing" and making facial grimaces.

After breakfast, the ranchers sit in the living room awaiting direction from Steven, the foreman, and assignments of morning chores. One of them tries to turn on the television, but it has been disconnected. The blaring talk, canned laughter, loud commercials, and rap music on television are prohibited during the day. The excessive stimulation, particularly in the morning, triggers chaotic behavior among the ranchers and can disrupt the relative calm and order of the ranch throughout the day.

Today, Mikey is to complete his usual chores of feeding hay to the two horses and filling the water trough. He and an aide walk to the barn, and Mikey automatically pulls a hay bale from the stack. It falls to the concrete floor, with dust billowing, causing Mikey to sneeze. The sneeze sets off several self-stimulating behaviors including rocking, repeatedly turning his head from left to right, and saying, "Dentist, dentist, dentist." The aide gently redirects Mikey to the stack of hay and points to another bale.

Mikey is not allowed to use sharp instruments unsupervised, and the aide gives him a brown pocket knife. Over the past few weeks, Mikey has learned to open it and safely cut the twine that is compressing the hay bale. Then he carefully closes the knife and says, "Dentist." Mikey enjoys this part of his chores and often needs coaxing to return the pocket knife to the aide.

One interesting aspect of Mikey's language is his tendency to confuse pronouns. This is apparent when the horses are fed and it is time to fill the water trough. Mikey turns to the aide and says, "You get hose." To the aide, it appears that Mikey wants him to put the hose in the water trough, but knowing Mikey's language, he realizes that the request is for Mikey to get the hose. The aide models the correct language construct and Mike correctly says, "Mikey get the hose now?" When the water trough is full, the two men return to the ranch house.

After the ranchers have completed their morning chores, they participate in individual and group occupational, physical, and speech therapies. Highly structured recreational activities are provided; the favorites are swimming and water games. After lunch, the ranchers have "quiet time" in their rooms or other parts of the ranch. Several ranchers play with the animals. There are rabbits, cats, dogs, chickens, horses, a pygmy goat, and Thomas, the huge turkey, who captivates the ranchers with his long neck and gobble. After the ranchers complete their evening chores, they have dinner and watch television or a video before bedtime. "Lights out" is at 9:00 p.m., but it usually takes longer for the ranchers to fall asleep, ending another day at Mikey's Moonshadow Ranch.

Case Study 1.4 Dysgraphia, Dyslexia, and an IEP Conference

ANDREW

Andrew's parents eagerly anticipate and also fear the approaching IEP conference about their only son. They eagerly wait to see what the public school professionals will do about his learning disability. They also fear that the tests will show that Andrew is mentally retarded and that there is little hope of his ever learning to write. Andrew has been struggling with writing for several years, and even now, in the fifth

Clinical Sidebar 1.4
The IEP details the services provided to children with disabilities. All IEPs should include the projected dates for initiation and duration of services, a statement of the child's present level of educational performance, short- and long-term goals, and criteria and evaluation procedures to determine whether the objectives are being met. They should also indicate the extent to which the child will be able to participate in regular classroom activities. What role should the child and his or her parents play in creating the IEP?

grade, he writes like a first grader. The IEP conference has been scheduled for 2 weeks, and as it approaches, their anxiety grows.

They enter the conference room, where the teachers and specialists are already sitting at a long wooden table. The conference coordinator is the director of special education, and she introduces them to the school psychologist, speech-language pathologist, and resource room teacher. Andrew's parents have already met his teacher, and they sit down at the conference table as the meeting begins. The coordinator explains the reason for the conference and reviews Andrew's problems with writing. Then she turns the meeting over to the school psychologist, who has done extensive intelligence and scholastic testing of Andrew.

The psychologist reviews the results of the intelligence test, one specifically designed for children, and reports that Andrew has a composite intelligence quotient of 136. Andrew's parents are relieved to find that the score is not only above average, it is high. The psychologist says that 136 is two standard deviations above the average for all persons, showing that Andrew is gifted. Then, seeing that the parents are not familiar with psychometrics and standard deviations, she explains that if persons who take intelligence tests are placed in similar groups, Andrew more closely resembles the small group of people who are above average in intelligence rather than those in the average group. The psychologist goes on to describe Andrew's strengths and weaknesses on the intelligence and scholastic tests. She concludes her report by saying that Andrew is a gifted student with learning disabilities.

The speech-language pathologist has also tested Andrew, and reports that not only does he have problems expressing himself in writing, he also has difficulties with reading. He notes that reading and writing problems often go hand-in-hand. Andrew's reading problem, dyslexia, is not nearly as severe as his writing deficit. Andrew will receive inclusion therapy in the classroom for these disorders, and the objectives for therapy will be blended into his academic curriculum. Although Andrew could receive individual or small-group therapy in the speech-language pathologist's office, inclusion therapy is recommended so that he can better achieve his literacy goals.

The resource teacher explains her role in helping Andrew. As her title indicates, she will serve as a resource for Andrew as he deals with his courses and learning disabilities. Andrew can leave his classroom and go to the resource room whenever he has difficulty completing an academic task. In addition, Andrew is scheduled for regular meetings with the resource teacher so that she can help him with written homework assignments. The resource teacher and the speech-language pathologist agree that Andrew is likely to overcome his writing problems without the aid of a speech-to-type device, in which a person speaks into an embedded microphone and the machine types what has been said while checking the grammar and spelling. Although some individuals with learning disabilities require this device to succeed in school, the team feels that Andrew can overcome his writing and reading disorders with the special services offered by the school.

Andrew's classroom teacher supports the special services that are available to him and discusses her role in helping him. She will encourage him to seek help from the resource teacher when needed and will adjust his assignments to accommodate his disability. For example, she will give Andrew more time to take written tests, allow him to take them in the resource room, and, when possible, permit oral examinations. She will also confer with the speech-language pathologist about integrating therapy goals with educational objectives.

According to the special education director, many children with learning disabilities discover new cognitive and learning styles to overcome their problems. Gifted children with learning disabilities often have unique ways of acquiring and internalizing information. Sometimes they can be very creative, turning a disability into an asset. The special education director reviews the short- and long-term objectives for Andrew and the criteria that will be used to measure his success in meeting them. She then turns the meeting over to Andrew's parents for questions, concerns, and comments.

Andrew's parents express their gratitude for the time the committee members have given to their son. They ask intelligent questions about the nature of the writing and reading problems, and whether it is likely that Andrew will ever be able to perform normally in school. They ask what caused the learning disabilities and how limiting they will be for Andrew throughout his life.

Members of the IEP team take turns answering the parents' questions. The speech-language pathologist reviews the nature of reading and writing problems and is optimistic. Andrew is likely to learn to write and read with only minimal accommodations in school. For the problems that do not resolve, he will be taught to compensate by developing alternate learning styles and skills. The team agrees that the causes of learning disabilities have yet to be discovered but that they likely involve differences in brain structure and/or chemistry. The entire team agrees that Andrew should prepare for college and that his learning disabilities will not be insurmountable obstacles. They explain that the Americans with Disabilities Act and the Individuals with Disabilities Education Act have opened many previously closed doors for persons with disabilities. They also note that technological advances have dramatically improved the lives of these people.

Case Study 1.5 Reporting Suspected Child Abuse in a Language-Delayed Preschooler

DAWN

The student clinician is excited about the midsemester conference she is to have with her supervisor. Dawn, a preschooler, is making remarkable gains in language therapy. She is small for her age, with beautiful dark eyes, and on rare occasions an ear-to-ear smile that brightens up the small therapy suite. She always wears conservative dresses, never shorts or jeans. Her parents are members of a religious group that also prohibits the cutting of hair, and Dawn's is either shaped into a bun or pony tail or hangs luxuriously from her head. The child has started to bond with the student clinician and eagerly anticipates therapy, obviously basking in the clinician's attention and affection.

During the initial sessions, it was hard to get Dawn to talk. When approached, the shy 4-year-old would turn her head and cry; she never initiated conversations. Gradually, Dawn is escaping her shell and is learning the pragmatics of language. A game called "Hi Ho Cherry O" is the key to Dawn's participation in therapy.

Dawn loves the game. Spinning the arrow, collecting the small red plastic cherries, and experiencing the thrill of winning by announcing, "Hi Ho Cherry O," provides a perfect means to improve Dawn's pragmatic language skills. During the game, the student clinician feigns ignorance of the rules and asks Dawn to explain how the game is played. Dawn is encouraged to engage in turn-taking and to maintain the topic of conversation. Usually she speaks in one- and two-word utterances, and the student clinician is working to increase their overall mean length. She is beginning to get Dawn to narrate her actions during the game and is making progress on additional communicative functions. However, she is troubled by the girl's frequent bruises and injuries.

Several times Dawn has come to the therapy session with large bruises on her arms and legs, and once, she sported a black-and-blue eye. When asked how she was injured, Dawn did not respond or simply said, "I fell down." Suspecting that the child was accident-prone, the clinician continued the therapy session. Recently, however, Dawn came to therapy with what appeared to be burns on her thighs, and the student clinician can no longer ignore the unthinkable. She asks her supervisor to look at Dawn's injuries. Afterward, they decide that the repeated injuries and the apparent burns warrant an investigation.

The university's Speech and Hearing Clinic has established a protocol for reporting child abuse. First, the student clinician must report suspected abuse to a supervisor. The supervisor is required to immediately file a report with the local office of Child Protective Services. Although the student clinician and the supervisor can question the child and parents about the source and nature of the injuries, they are not to investigate them or to indicate their suspicion of child abuse. Child Protective Services sends a social worker to the family's home to investigate the complaint. The identity of the complainants is kept anonymous to prevent retaliation. If the social worker believes there are grounds for further investigation of child abuse and/or that the child's health or safety is in jeopardy, a court order is obtained and the child is immediately placed in temporary foster care as a ward of the state. The student clinician and the supervisor know the significance and implications of their actions, but they are morally, ethically, and legally bound to report any suspected child abuse. They also realize that it is not their responsibility to prove the abuse, only to report it if they believe the child is in imminent danger.

Clinical Sidebar 1.5

Speech and hearing professionals see thousands of children annually; consequently, they are likely to encounter child abuse. Because of the heinous and abhorrent nature of crimes against children, it is natural for professionals not to suspect that a child is being abused. However, speech and hearing professionals are legally, morally, and ethically required to immediately report suspected child abuse to the proper officials. What procedures would you follow if you suspected that a child was being abused at home?

The suspected child abuse was confirmed by the investigating social worker. Dawn was removed from her home and placed with foster parents. Child Protective Services was careful to disrupt only minimally Dawn's preschool activities and her therapy at the Speech and Hearing Clinic. Also, to provide continuity, there would be no change in the student clinician at the end of the semester. The social worker met with the supervisor and the student clinician to discuss the case, and offered helpful suggestions in dealing with Dawn should she question or want to talk about the separation from her parents. Without providing details about the abuse or how long it had continued, the social worker thanked the supervisor and the student clinician for their professionalism in reporting it. The social worker commented that, tragically, the severity of child abuse often escalates, and that their prompt reporting of it may have saved Dawn from greater trauma.

Case Study **1.6**   Severe Mental Impairment–Mental Retardation in a 2-Year-Old

ELIZABETH

It is nearly a 3-hour drive to the small community in the northwest corner of the state. Many of the townspeople belong to a sect noted for plural marriages, an offshoot of a major religion that long ago disallowed polygamy. Curiously, the state seems to turn a blind eye to the region's polygamy, possibly to avoid a head-on collision concerning the separation of church and state. You, as a consultant to the state's Department of Developmental Disabilities, have been asked to evaluate a child with multiple birth defects and severe mental retardation. The agency wants to know if she is capable of learning language. The social worker was succinct: "What, if anything, can be done to help her learn to communicate?" The officials are considering removing the child from the care of her grandmother and institutionalizing her.

As you drive through the small town, you become increasingly aware that you are a stranger to the tight-knit community. People on the sidewalk stare relentlessly as you search for the home in the maze of unlabeled streets. You note that all of the women wear dresses typical of early pioneers and that there is no shortage of children. Finally, you find the correct address and pull into the gravel driveway of an ancient two-story brick home. Later, you learn that homes like this were built to accommodate bigamous marriages. There are two separate kitchens, living rooms, bathrooms, and bedrooms. You are greeted by a woman in her 50s, the grandmother of the child you are to evaluate. Apparently, the child's mother was living in Los Angeles and returned home soon after the child was born. She has since left the community and abandoned her child. The grandmother expresses her sorrow about her daughter's decision but says that she is happy to care for her granddaughter. You see the 2-year-old in a homemade crib and are startled at the severity of her defects. Reading the case history did not prepare you for the reality.

According to her grandmother, Elizabeth was born almost 2 months prematurely. Her mother may have tried to induce an abortion, was a heavy user of alcohol and drugs, and was in a drunken stupor during most of her pregnancy and when

Elizabeth was born. The grandmother continued the litany of birth defects, confirming the medical reports. Elizabeth is deaf, partially paralyzed on the right side of her body, almost completely blind, and in need of several operations to correct her deformed spine. The medical reports suggest that Elizabeth had probably suffered a stroke during the pregnancy.

Clinical Sidebar 1.6
Sometimes it is difficult to directly assess cognitive, linguistic, and social-communication development in a child with multiple severe disabilities. Indirect assessment using parents or guardians as knowledgeable informants can provide valuable information about a child's acquisition and use of language. They should be questioned in non-technical terms and clinical jargon avoided. Why do some speech-language pathologists believe that parents are inaccurate or mistaken when evaluating their children's mental development?

When you ask about the 2-year-old's communication abilities, you discover that she has differential crying and that her grandmother can tell from the loudness, pitch, and tone of the cry whether she is hungry, in pain, needs a diaper change, and so forth. Elizabeth cries at an appropriate volume and does not appear to have laryngeal paralysis. She cooed at a normal age and began babbling. However, no further language development has been observed. Elizabeth's face and tongue are paralyzed on the right side, and she requires special and frequent feeding using a syringe. The psychological reports suggest that she has profound mental impairment—mental retardation, and although a firm determination cannot be made due to her hearing and visual impairments, her intelligence quotient is thought to be between 30 and 40. You do as many tests as possible to get some idea of Elizabeth's language mental age, strengths, and weaknesses.

You are no stranger to the terrible injuries and birth defects afflicting humans, having seen hundreds of cases in which the patient's likelihood of ever having a reasonable quality of life is remote. But the plight of this young, innocent child, and the severity of her multiple birth defects, nearly brings tears to your eyes. Her condition seems so unfair, her future so compromised, and her disabilities so insurmountable.

You spend most of the day with Elizabeth and her grandmother, watching their interaction. The grandmother is an intelligent, caring, energetic, and nurturing woman. Elizabeth seems to require constant care, and her grandmother provides it. At Elizabeth's first sound, her grandmother automatically attends to her, almost as if they communicate telepathically. Although Elizabeth is deaf, her grandmother talks to her while caressing, soothing, and comforting her. Their interaction is natural and unstrained. Occasionally, the grandmother gets irritated at a messy diaper and baby food pushed aside, but nevertheless, she is loving and caring. You marvel at her dedication, commitment, and devotion to this abandoned child.

On the drive home, you mentally prepare the report you will write to the Department of Developmental Disabilities. As a realist, you know that the likelihood of Elizabeth's ever communicating functionally is remote, even with the most experienced therapists and the best technology. In fact, there are no speech-language pathologists within 100 miles of Elizabeth's town, and regular individual and group therapies are unobtainable while she lives with grandmother. If the state institutionalizes her, a multitude of therapies will be available. She will have all the services required by state and federal laws, including regular aural rehabilitation, as well as speech and language therapy. As a realist, you also know that what is legally obtainable for the child will not be best for her.

In your report to the agency, you make clear recommendations for Elizabeth and speech-language pathology services. You state that from a communication development standpoint, training the child's grandmother in language development is preferable to removing the child from her loving home and institutionalizing her. You review the test results showing that Elizabeth has profound language delay, and you report that the prognosis for functional language development is poor. Certainly, there are areas where Elizabeth can improve, as well as devices and therapies that may help her to achieve her maximum potential. You recommend that the agency contract with a speech-language pathologist to visit Elizabeth weekly, work with her grandmother to maximize communication, provide individual therapy, and set realistic goals. Several months later, the agency reports that you, and virtually all of the other consultants, have agreed that Elizabeth was already receiving the best possible services from her grandmother. Rather than remove the child from her loving environment, the agency will use all of its resources to support her grandmother in the care of this child.

Case Study **1.7** Language Therapy in a Teenager with Down Syndrome

ELROY

In many ways, Elroy is a typical teenager. That he was born with Down syndrome does not detract from his teenage ways. In fact, his easygoing, pleasant personality, typical of individuals with this chromosome disorder, is an antidote to the surly ways of many 17-year-old boys. Elroy still has the typical male teenage angst, aggressiveness, and misdirected energy, but he seems more responsible than many of his peers.

Clinical Sidebar 1.7
Down syndrome is also known as *trisomy 21 syndrome* because it is characterized by chromosome 21 irregularities. What are the physical and mental characteristics of persons with this syndrome?

Elroy works in a sheltered environment. Friendship Industries employs many teenagers and adults with special needs, and at this shop there are three persons with Down syndrome. At 17, Elroy is one of the youngest employees, and he has worked there for 4 years. He is assigned to the Day Old Bread Store. Teddy's Bread Company, a local bakery and distributor of breads and pastries to grocery stores, restaurants, and fast-food establishments, generously donates to Friendship Industries their older and nearly stale bakery products. They are sold in a small freestanding red building on the grounds of the sheltered workshop. The products sold in the store are discounted by more than half of their retail price, and many people in the community purchase bread there. Occasionally, customers return a loaf of bread when they discover spots of green mold, but usually they are satisfied.

Twice a week, two student clinicians and their supervisor from the university come to Friendship Industries to provide speech and language therapy to the employees. Elroy's student clinician works on language pragmatics, counting change, and teaching him to follow the instructions on how to rotate the loaves of bread. Elroy is having trouble with the concept of bread rotation. Each loaf of bread is sealed with a small colored tab. Few customers realize that the color of the tab indicates when the loaf was baked. These tabs tell the bread distributor when a loaf of bread is getting old and needs to be pulled from the shelves. They also tell Elroy what loaves should be at the front of the shelf so that the oldest bread is sold first, reducing the number of loaves that need to be discarded.

Elroy has learned to count change well enough to work behind the counter, even during the busiest times. Largely due to what he has learned in language therapy, he carefully computes the change customers receive. The clinicians taught him how to use the cash register and to double-check his figures. Only once has a customer reported being short-changed, and the supervisor found that Elroy was correct. Another customer complained about how long it took to serve her, but Elroy's slow, meticulous handling of money is encouraged.

The student clinicians are teaching Elroy to follow written instructions for bread rotation. They have given him a laminated sheet of paper showing which day the bread was baked and the color of the tab that denotes it. To help Elroy understand bread rotation, the clinicians have placed colored marks on a large calendar. In language therapy, they have taught Elroy to examine the calendar to learn the day of the week. Once this is determined, he notes the color mark next to it. Although Elroy knows the colors, it has taken him several months to learn the relationship between the numbers on the calendar and the days of the week. Now that he has mastered the calendar, the clinicians have written on another laminated sheet of paper: "If today is 'blue,' then 'black' should be at the front of the shelf. If today is 'yellow,' then 'purple' should be at the front of the shelf." Each rotation schedule is identified accordingly. In addition, the words referring to colors are written in appropriately colored ink, and the procedure is illustrated.

Today, Elroy is "going solo," as the clinicians call it. He has achieved all of the therapy objectives in the clinical situation, and now he is to put into practice his hard-won education about bread rotation. With both clinicians trailing him, Elroy walks to the Day Old Bread Store. A new delivery of bread has recently arrived, and in the stock room he sorts the loaves onto trays by the color of the tabs. He looks to the clinicians for approval, which is given by a thumbs-up gesture. Then Elroy carries the trays to the front of the store. After examining the laminated sheets of paper and the calendar, he carefully places the loaves of bread on the shelves. Soon, all of the loaves on the shelves are properly rotated, and Elroy beams with satisfaction. The stale bread is taken to the disposal area, where a local farmer will give it to his pigs. Apparently, the pigs do not care if there is a little green mold on their food.

SUMMARY

Persons with disordered or delayed language are at a distinct disadvantage; language is necessary to succeed in school, vocation, and relationships. In addition, language and thought are fundamentally related, and there are certain cognitive prerequisites to learning and using language. Many language disorders are associated with learning disabilities, and speech-language pathologists are taking an ever-increasing leadership role in children's literacy development. Federal, state, and local laws and regulations dictate the special education services provided to individuals with language delay and disorders.

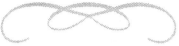

Study and Discussion Questions

1. Provide your own definition of language.

2. What are the modalities of language and the learning disabilities affecting them?

3. How does a symbol differ from an image?

4. Describe the relationship between language and thought.

5. What are cognitive prerequisites, and what role do they play in language acquisition?

6. Describe the differences between language competence and language performance.

7. Describe the typical communication behaviors of a child with pragmatic language deficits.

8. Define and describe dyslexia.

9. Define and describe dysgraphia.

10. What are some of the language problems seen in persons with autism, attentional deficit disorders, and mental impairment–mental retardation?

11. What is IDEA, and how does it relate to the treatment of language delay and disorders?

12. Provide an example of how a person's culture may affect language testing.

Recommended Reading

Kagan, S., and Kagan, M. (1998). *Multiple intelligences: The complete MI book*. San Clemente, CA: Kagan Cooperative Learning.

This book proposes and describes eight types of multiple intelligences.

Tanner, D. (2003). *The forensic aspects of communication sciences and disorders*. Tucson, AZ: Lawyers and Judges.

Several chapters in this book address the legal ramifications of providing special education services and include references to published legal cases.

CHAPTER TWO

Articulation and Phonology Disorders

When I was a child, I spake as a child, I understood as a child, I thought as a child; but when I became a man I put away childish things.

1 Corinthians 13:11

Chapter Preview: This chapter addresses the human ability to make speech sounds and the disorders that can occur. Articulatory structures, anatomy and physiology, phonetics, and phonology are reviewed. Children's acquisition of speech sounds is discussed, as are dialect and accent. Articulation and phonology disorders are reviewed in terms of their etiology, diagnosis, and treatment. Case studies are presented involving lisping, /w/ for /r/ substitution, multiple articulation errors, group therapy, and appropriate use of augmentative and alternative communication devices.

OVERVIEW OF ARTICULATION AND PHONOLOGY DISORDERS

When used in speech sound production, the word **articulate** means to combine the movements of two or more oral structures into speech sounds. **Articulation** involves shaping compressed air from the lungs into individual speech sounds; the vocal tract structures are moved so that speech sounds are produced. There are two ways of viewing these speech disorders. In the **traditional approach**, articulation disorders are considered structural and functional deficits involving the articulators and impairments in learning the sensory, motor, and perceptual features associated with speech sound production. Phonology is the rule-governed way humans produce the sounds of language. In the **phonological approach**, speech sound production disorders are viewed as delayed acquisition of the phonological rules of the language. To treat the communication disorder, the clinician helps the child discover adult phonology. Although these two approaches to speech production disorders appear significantly different in etiology and treatment, they overlap and are similar. There is a strong relationship between the discovery of phonological processes and traditional phoneme acquisition (Culbertson & Tanner, 2001a), on the one hand, and dependence of neuromotor oral maturation on phonological development, on the other (Culbertson & Tanner, 2001b).

Articulatory Anatomy and Physiology

The articulators can be divided into **fixed** and **mobile** and **soft** and **hard**. The primary fixed articulators are the hard palate, alveolar ridge, and upper incisors. The mobile articulators are the tongue, velum (soft palate), mandible, and lips. The main soft articulators are the lips, tongue, and velum, and the primary hard articulators are the teeth, mandible, hard palate, and alveolar ridge. Figure 2.1 shows the human articulators.

As Figure 2.1 shows, the hard palate extends across the top of the oral cavity. The palatal vault is the dome-shaped top part of the oral cavity and houses the resting tongue. The palatal vault can be considered high, medium, or low, and in most persons it has a discernible shape: trapezoid, triangular, or oval. The positioning of the tongue relative to the palatal vault gives most speech sounds, especially vowels, their distinctive acoustic qualities. The alveolar ridge, the tissue just behind the upper incisors at the front (anterior) of the hard palate, is an important articulatory structure for the production of several consonants (see below). For example, the tip of the tongue contacts the alveolar ridge in the production of /t/, /d/, and /l/ sounds. It and the tongue are also important points of articulatory constriction for the /s/ and sh sounds. The upper incisors are a point of contact for the tongue and for the constriction of the airstream in the production of several phonemes, such as the voiced and voiceless th. The lips open and close in the production of bilabials such as /b/ and /m/ and have various degrees of rounding, giving vowels their distinctive acoustic qualities. The lower lip and the upper incisors approximate each other in the production of phonemes such as /v/ and /f/.

The human tongue is the most important articulator and consists of the root, base, and blade. **Intrinsic** tongue muscles have their origin and attachment within the tongue. These muscles primarily shape the tongue for speech and **mastication** (chewing). **Extrinsic** tongue muscles have their attachment outside the tongue and are primarily involved in moving it. According to Ladefoged and Maddieson (1988), there are approximately 16 different places of consonant articulation in the world's languages.

Phonetics

In the mid-1800s, scientists created the **International Phonetic Alphabet** (IPA). One reason was to make the labeling of speech sounds consistent. In English, 26 letters can be used for labeling the 44 phonemes of the language. Obviously, this creates situations in which some **graphemes** (letters) must be used for more than one sound and vice versa. Ideally, the speech sound, the **phoneme**, should always be represented by one and only one letter. The IPA provides for that phoneme-grapheme equality. It also specifies the acoustic and perceptual features of each phoneme. Figure 2.2 shows the IPA grapheme for each phoneme and provides examples of pronunciation.

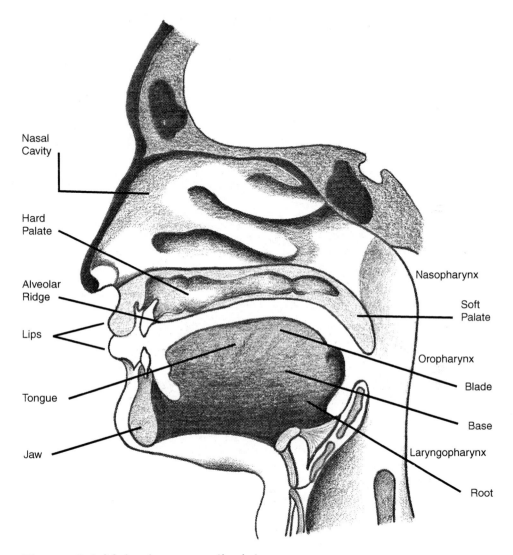

Figure 2.1 Major human articulators.

Consonants

There are two ways consonant phonemes can be classified: by **place** and by **manner** of production. In classification by place, consonants are categorized by where in the oral cavity they are produced. The **glottal** phoneme /h/ is produced at the level of the vocal cords, and the **lingua-velar** site is the tongue and soft palate. **Lingua-palatal**, **lingua-alveolar**, and **lingua-dental** sites are the tongue and palate, tongue and alveolar ridge, and tongue

Consonants			
p	as pronounced in the word pin	m	as pronounced in the word milk
h	as pronounced in the word hurt	ð	as pronounced in the word that
v	as pronounced in the word vast	k	as pronounced in the word climb
f	as pronounced in the word food	l	as pronounced in the word lamb
θ	as pronounced in the word think	g	as pronounced in the word gone
ʃ	as pronounced in the word shoot	z	as pronounced in the word zipper
n	as pronounced in the word no	ŋ	as pronounced in the word sing
t	as pronounced in the word tag	b	as pronounced in the word button
d	as pronounced in the word do	dʒ	as pronounced in the word jump
s	as pronounced in the word so	j	as pronounced in the word yellow
w	as pronounced in the word water	tʃ	as pronounced in the word chicken
r	as pronounced in the word rabbit	ʒ	as pronounced in the word beige

Vowels			
U	as pronounced in the word book	ɛ	as pronounced in the word head
ɝ	as pronounced in the word bird	o	as pronounced in the word over
I	as pronounced in the word his	ʌ	as pronounced in the word mother
ɑ	as pronounced in the word top	ɔ	as pronounced in the word tall
æ	as pronounced in the word cat	u	as pronounced in the word you
i	as pronounced in the word see	e	as pronounced in the word ache

Figure 2.2 IPA symbols and examples of pronunciation.

and teeth articulatory sites, respectively. **Labio-dentals** are sounds produced at the lips and teeth, and **bilabials** are produced by the action of both lips.

In categorization by the manner the airstream is shaped into speech sounds, consonants are divided into two categories: **stops** and **continuants**. Stops involve the complete cessation of the airstream and acoustic energy, while continuants have continuous airflow during their production. **Nasals** involve increased nasal resonance due to the opening of the velopharyngeal port, and **glides** require movement of the articulators. **Fricatives** are produced by constriction of the airstream, and **plosives** have an abrupt explosion of air. **Affricates** are explosions of air shaped into continuants. A **blend** is two or more consonants without a vowel separating them, sometimes called a **consonant cluster**.

Vowels

All vowels are voiced and depend on the **height** and **front-to-back** position of the tongue in the oral cavity. For example, some vowels are classified as **low-back**, **high-front**, **high-back**, and so on, depending on the tongue's prominence in the oral cavity. **Lip rounding** also plays a role in their acoustic qualities. A **diphthong** is produced by moving the articulators from one vowel articulatory position to another. The vowel is central to the **syllable**, a unit of speech having a vowel as its central physiological and acoustic property. The types of syllables are represented using *V* for vowel and *C* for consonant, for example, CV (*be*), CVC (*bun*), VC (*up*), and CCV (*sleigh*).

Coarticulation and Assimilation

Rarely do people produce individual speech sounds in isolation (**static articulation**) unconnected to strings of other phonemes. Most speech sounds are produced in rapid succession as part of longer utterances (**dynamic speech**). Oral movements during dynamic articulation occur very rapidly, involving more than 100 muscles and thousands of neurological impulses per second. Because of the rapid movement of the articulators during speech, units of speech run into each other. As a result, articulatory movements only approximate their ideal points of contact. In dynamic utterances, speech sounds become more like each other. **Coarticulation** is the overlapping of articulatory movements during dynamic speech. **Assimilation** is the effect that one sound has on another. Coarticulation leads to assimilation.

Phonology

Whereas the sensorimotor approach to articulation development and disorders considers speech sound learning as a product of auditory perception and the development of fine motor skills, the phonological approach involves language. **Phonology** is the rule-governed way humans produce the sounds of language. It is one aspect of language, the others being semantics, syntax, and grammar. When an individual has a phonologically based articulation disorder, learning the phonological rules is the treatment objective. Rather than teach the production of one and only one sound, clinicians use several sounds to teach the rules of phonology.

In the phonological approach to articulation development and disorders, speech sound development is considered the **discovery** and **fusion** of syllable formation principles. In this approach, articulation disorders are thought to result from delayed acquisition of the **phonological rules** of the language. Phonological rules or **processes** are simplified linguistic behaviors used by children when they attempt to produce adult speech. To treat a communication disorder, the clinician helps the child discover adult phonology. More than one sound is used to teach the phonological rules. This approach is particularly useful for children who have more than one articulation disorder and for those with impaired intelligibility. Figure 2.3 shows **syllable structure**, **substitution**, and **harmony processes** and their ages of normal **extinction** (Tanner, Culbertson, & Secord, 1997).

Phoneme Acquisition Ages

As Figure 2.4 shows, the sequence of phoneme acquisition in children is relatively **invariant**, whereas the rate is highly **variable**. In all languages, **phonetic duplications** are the most common types of first words. In English, most children's first words are phonetic duplications such as *mama* and *dada*. According to Tanner et al. (1997), 75% of children have acquired the following phonemes in all positions of words (initial, medial, final) by age 3 years: /m/, /h/, /w/, /n/, *ng,* and /f/. Seventy-five percent of children have acquired the phonemes /ʒ/ and /ð/ in all three positions of words by age 7 years. Consequently, 75% of

COMPOSITE AGES OF NORMAL PHONOLOGICAL PROCESS EXTINCTION

Instructions: Draw a heavy horizontal line at the child's age level for comparison purposes.

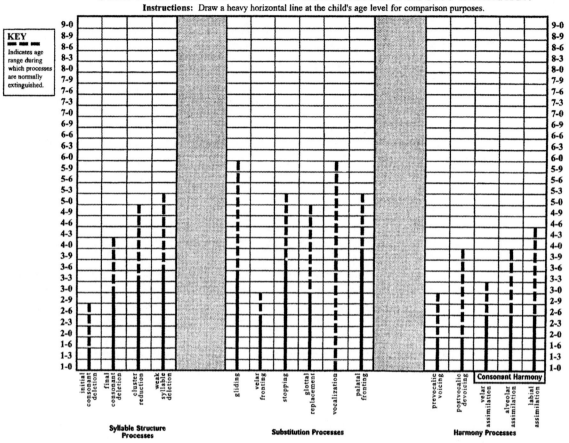

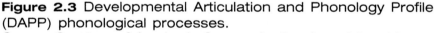

Figure 2.3 Developmental Articulation and Phonology Profile (DAPP) phonological processes.
Source: Courtesy of Academic Communication Associates. May not be reproduced without written permission of the publisher.

children learn to produce the phonemes of English in the **initial**, **medial**, and **final** positions of words between 3 and 7 years of age. The two most common misarticulated consonant phonemes, /r/ and /s/, are established at 4 years, 6 months and 4 years, 9 months, respectively, by 75% of children in all three positions of words.

Errors in Articulation

Although children may **substitute**, **distort**, **add**, and **omit** vowels during speech production, the most common articulatory errors involve consonants. Vowels and diphthongs are

CONSONANT DEVELOPMENT CHART

Instructions: Draw a heavy horizontal line at the child's age level for comparison purposes.

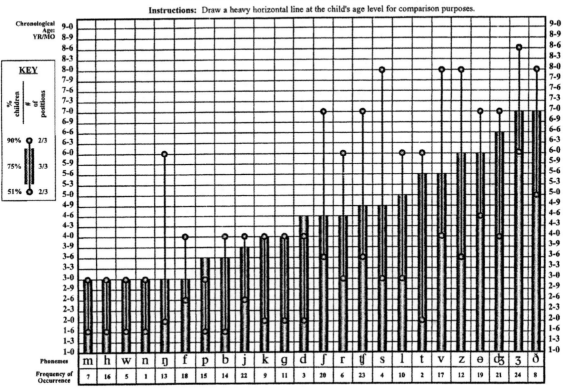

Figure 2.4 DAPP consonants.

Source: Courtesy of Academic Communication Associates. May not be reproduced without written permission of the publisher.

mastered by most children before the age of 4 years (Tanner et al., 1997). Phoneme acquisition sequence and rate may also have minor variance by geographic region, for example, Northern versus Southern states. Why are vowels more likely to be produced correctly and consonants misarticulated by children? Four acoustic, physiological, and perceptual factors can account for this difference.

First, vowels are less likely to be misarticulated because all vowels are voiced. Voicing gives phonemes greater acoustic energy and sends the listener more perceptual features about their production. Second, vowels are less complicated to articulate than consonants. Although fine tongue and lip-rounding movements are necessary to produce vowels, consonants typically require more articulatory excursions, making them more vulnerable to misarticulation. Third, vowels are the core of the syllable, so their acoustic, physiological, and perceptual features are more conspicuous and salient. Finally, as a group, vowels occur more frequently than consonants, giving the person

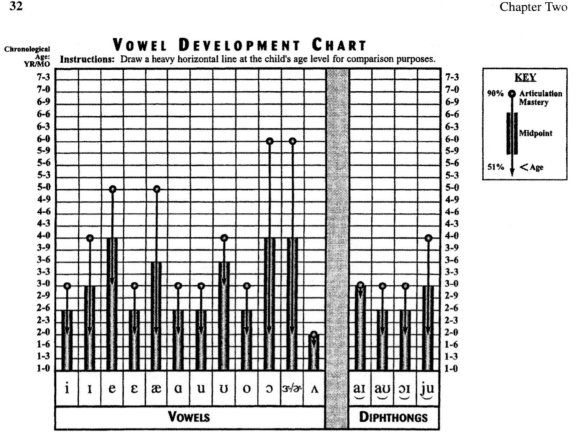

Figure 2.5 DAPP vowels.
Source: Courtesy of Academic Communication Associates. May not be reproduced without written permission of the publisher.

more opportunities to learn them. Figure 2.5 shows the ages at which vowels and diphthongs are mastered.

Accent and Dialect

Accents and **dialects** are more varied in the eastern United States because that is where many immigrants first settled (Alvarez & Kolker, 1987). These terms are often used interchangeably, but technically they differ. An accent indicates the articulation traits of the speaker's first learned language carried over to a second acquired language. A dialect is a specific pronunciation and vocabulary used in a particular geographical area and socioeconomic stratum and can include an accent. There are no substandard accents and dialects; all rule-governed cultural variations in the production and use of speech and language are normal.

Accent and dialect are **nonstandard**, not **substandard**, speech and language. They are examples of complex linguistic variations and social adaption. Wolfram (1986) comments on the complexities of these linguistic variations:

> One of the ironies of our understanding of linguistic variation is the fact that this complex behavior has so often been reduced to simplistic and uninformed explanation, being attributed to ignorance and simplicity. Nothing could be farther from the truth; instead, linguistic variation deserves our utmost respect as a representation of the complex workings of the human mind and human social adaptive mechanism. (p. 114)

Accent and dialect also suggest a speaker's ethnicity, culture, religion, socioeconomic status, and homeland and can be useful in **speaker profiling** for forensic purposes (Tanner & Tanner, 2004). Speaker profiling is the forensic information obtained from accent and dialect, indicating homeland and ethnicity. It can be used to prevent terrorist attacks. Speaker profiling is not the same as racial profiling. Although some speakers may want accent and dialect reduction by speech-language pathologists, accent and dialect variations are not speech pathologies. Thus, accent and dialect reduction are not covered by insurance companies or provided as standard speech pathology services by public schools. Persons seeking this therapy do so for personal, professional, and occupational reasons or because of reduced intelligibility.

Etiology of Articulation Disorders

There are several causal factors in articulation and phonology disorders. In the past, the **etiology** of articulation disorders was not an important factor in diagnosing and treating them because few therapies existed. Today, however, etiology has become an important factor in selecting diagnostic protocols and planning treatment. Articulation disorders may be caused by deafness, hearing loss, structural abnormalities, neuromuscular impairments, delayed language, emotional duress, and neuromotor maturation inadequacies.

Deafness and Hearing Loss

Children acquire the sounds and phonology of the language to which they are exposed. For example, children reared by Navajo, Hopi, Japanese, or Spanish speakers learn the speech sounds and phonology of those languages. Children born deaf do not normally acquire any true speech sounds or phonology because they are deprived of the auditory exposure required to learn them. These children have undifferentiated and differentiated crying, cooing, and begin the babbling stage at the same time as hearing children. However, without special intervention or therapies, children who are deaf do not progress beyond this stage and learn speech. Of course, the age at which a child loses his or her hearing is important in determining what level of articulation and phonology intervention is necessary. An older child with hearing loss will have heard speech sounds and will probably have learned them.

The effect of partial hearing loss on articulation and phonological development also depends on the age when it occurs. Similar to a child who is deaf, a child who loses his or her hearing before the age of approximately 7 or 8 years may have been exposed to the auditory stimulation necessary to learn speech sounds and phonology. Infants born **hard-of-hearing** have greater difficulty learning the phonemes and phonological structures of language than children who lose their hearing later in life. In addition, the frequency of the hearing loss must be considered. Some hearing disorders primarily involve the higher, middle, or lower frequency ranges, causing particular phonemes to be more distorted. For example, a child with a prominently high frequency hearing loss is likely to misarticulate speech sounds such as /s/, *sh,* and /z/ while mastering lower frequency speech sounds such as *ah,* /w/, and /l/.

Structural Abnormalities

Any defect, malformation, deformity, or irregularity of the oral structures can impair articulation. These structural abnormalities impair or prohibit the excursion, contact, and mobility of the articulators during speech. The severity of the articulatory disorders is usually related to the extent of the structural defects.

   Cleft lip and palate also affects articulation. In these **congenital birth defects** there is incomplete fusion of the lips, palatal shelves, and velum. Consequently, the articulators may be impaired or unable to create the airstream valving necessary for normal speech. Individuals with bilateral, complete clefts usually have more impaired articulation. Individuals with cleft palate, and those with dental and orthodontic impairments, may also have prematurely missing or jumbled teeth, causing the production of dental phonemes to be distorted.

   Some individuals have disproportionately large or small tongues and/or palatal vaults that are insufficient to house them properly. A disproportionately large tongue, **macroglossia**, occurs more frequently in persons with Down syndrome, resulting in slowly produced, distorted speech. Tongue reduction surgery is sometimes used to counter the effects of the macroglossia. A disproportionately small tongue, **microglossia**, is rare but can also reduce the precision of speech. Also rare is a shortened **lingual frenulum**, a cord of tissue running from the floor of the mouth to the middle of the underside of the tongue. In some children, the lingual frenulum may be too short to give the tongue functional mobility, especially the necessary elevation for phonemes such as /t/, /d/, and *th.* The lingual frenulum must be excised or "clipped" to permit proper mobility.

   Other structural abnormalities include partial or complete **glossectomy**, surgical removal of the tongue, usually because of oral cancer treatment. In automobile accidents and other high speed impacts, a victim may be thrust forward and bite off the tongue tip. Oral-facial anomalies affecting the size and positioning of the mandible in relation to the maxilla may also result in structural articulation disorders.

Neuromuscular Impairments

Two types of neurological impairments can affect articulation: **apraxia of speech** and the **dysarthrias**. Although both types often occur in aphasia, they are motor, not language, communication disorders. In motor speech disorders, articulation, one of the five basic motor speech processes, can be impaired by the neurological damage.

   Apraxia of speech primarily affects articulation and is a disorder of **speech programming**. The **articulatory plan**, consisting of all of the articulatory movements necessary to produce an utterance is disrupted. Although it can affect voluntary movements of the lips and velum, the tongue is primarily affected. The articulatory plan may be formulated in several areas of the brain, including the anterior insula and lateral premotor cortex (Wise, Greene, Büchel, & Scott, 1999). In apraxia of speech, this plan may be disrupted at the **conceptual level**, where the speaker is unable to discern the idea or concept driving the speech act. The speaker is impaired or unable to articulate due to ideational apraxia. Apraxia of speech may also impair articulation at the **planning level**, where the tongue's timing, speed, and strength are determined. Finally, apraxia of speech may disrupt the **activation of the neural commands** to the muscles of the tongue.

The dysarthrias are neurogenic communication disorders arising from muscular paralysis and/or an imbalance/deficiency of neurotransmitters. When the dysarthrias affect the articulatory valve, the type of paralysis determines the effects on articulation. **Lower motor neuron** involvement results in **flaccid** paralysis, in which the articulatory muscles have reduced tone. **Bilateral upper motor neuron** damage causes **spastic** articulatory muscles, with excessive tone and limited excursions. Damage to the **cerebellar system** causes the articulatory muscles to be jerky, ill-coordinated, and inefficient in producing voluntary speech movements. The articulatory errors in **ataxic** dysarthria are usually inconsistent. Disorders of the **extrapyramidal** motor system affect articulation in two ways. First, **hypokinesis** causes rigidity, reduced range of articulatory movement, diminished stress, and imprecise articulation. Second, **hyperkinesis** results in involuntary articulatory movements such as muscular tics and jerks. These movements result in interjections of grunts and other unwanted sounds during speech.

Delayed Language

One way of determining whether a child has a communication disorder is to compare the child's **chronological age** with his or her **mental age**. (The other way is to look at the child's **functional** communication abilities in everyday interactions.) Chronological age is the number of years and months the child has been alive. Mental age, also expressed in years and months, is a measure of the child's intelligence, or some other category of cognitive functioning and maturation, relative to established age norms. When a child's chronological age is significantly greater than his or her mental age on some parameter of language competence or performance, the child is consider to have language delay. Children who have phonological delay have not acquired the phonological systems of their peers.

Children whose test scores indicate that they have mental impairment–mental retardation often have delayed phonological development. For example, an individual with a tested mental age of 2 years, regardless of chronological age, is likely to have the phoneme acquisition and phonological process of a toddler. There are exceptions because of the variability of acquisition rates (see above) and because some children have unusually sophisticated fine motor development. However, as a rule, a child's mental age is indicative of his or her phonology acquisition potential.

Emotional Duress

There are etiological forms of stuttering, voice disorders, and deafness resulting from psychological and emotional factors. They are well-established clinical entities and are usually based on **hysteria** and **conversion reactions**. In these psychological phenomena, the physical disorder originates in a psychological conflict or repressed need. Often the physical disorder characterizes the conflict or psychological need, and patients are said to have a *symptom choice;* their symptoms **symbolize** the conflict or need. Loss of speech and hearing suggests interpersonal conflicts or impoverished communication. Articulation delay and regression also may be psychological in etiology and are usually classified as **elective mutism** or **idiopathic** articulation disorders.

Normal children do not regress significantly in articulation development; a 5-year-old does not normally use the speech of a toddler. When significant regression occurs, it is usually neurologically based or a result of psychological trauma. The psychological trauma may be the loss of a loved one through divorce, separation, or death, or because of neglect and abuse. A period of **mutism** often precedes regression of speech and language abilities that is typical of hysterical stuttering (Van Riper, 1992). The regression in speech articulation is related to the child's return to a more secure and comfortable psychological state, with speech patterns reflecting that coping style and defense mechanism. In children with speech articulation disorders related to emotional stress, treatment should also include a psychological referral, and reports to an appropriate social agency in cases of suspected neglect and abuse.

Neuromotor Maturation Inadequacies

In the phonological approach to articulation disorders, the child **simplifies** adult phonology and is delayed in learning age-appropriate phonological rules. "In his or her attempts to use language, the child in effect makes systematic simplifications of the phonology. From this point of view, children with a phonological disorder continue to use a simplification process beyond the time when others [of] their age use them" (Plante & Beeson, 2004, p. 65). In the phonological approach, the child with articulation errors has a delay, in contrast to a child with an articulation disorder.

Sensorimotor articulation inadequacies, as described here, refer to children who have one or two articulation disorders and have not mastered those particular phonemes at age-appropriate times. Isolated **lisping** and **/w/ for /r/ substitutions** are typical sensorimotor articulation errors that can be viewed not as a larger phonological disorder, but as an impairment or deficiency in auditory perception and in learning fine oral-motor speech skills. However, the articulation disorders originally may have been part of a larger phonological disorder and a simplification of adult phonology; the two theories are not mutually exclusive. Culbertson and Tanner (2001a, 2001b) have shown the strong relationship between neuromotor maturation and phonological development. Because of auditory perceptual and oral-motor habit strength, many children who lisp and have isolated /w/ for /r/ substitutions simply need traditional articulation therapy, not global phonology development therapies.

Diagnosing Articulation and Phonology Disorders

Diagnosing articulation and phonology disorders is sometimes called the **three-by-three** system. In this system, three types of articulatory errors are identified in the **initial**, **medial**, and **final** positions of syllables and words: **omissions**, **distortions**, and **substitutions**.

An omission is the deletion or neglect of a particular phoneme that should occur in a syllable or word. For example, a child may say __*at* for "cat" or __*ee* for "see". In phonology, omissions occur as part of changes in the structure of the syllable when the child simplifies speech by omitting a phoneme or phonemes. For example, omissions occur with cluster reduction, deletion of final or initial consonants, deletion of unstressed syllables, and syllable reduction. Clinicians identify omission on the record sheet by writing "om" where the phoneme should occur.

A distortion is the substitution of a nonstandard phoneme. The child produces a sound not recognized in his or her language system (however, it may be a recognizable phoneme in another language). Increasingly severe distortions are recorded as D_1, D_2, and D_3, respectively. A nasal distortion, in which there is audible escape of air through the child's nose (nasal emission), or hypernasality is identified as *D-nasal.*

Substitutions are identified by the required phoneme and the one that replaces it. For example, using the /w/ phoneme in place of the desired /r/ speech sound is written "w/r," and the position of the syllable or word is also indicated. A client who lisps in the middle of words (θ/s, medially) may be described as having a "/θ/ for /s/ substitution in the medial position." There are several phonological processes involving substitutions, including gliding of fricatives, in which a glide is replaced by a fricative, and stopping, in which a fricative is replaced by a stop consonant.

Additions are insertions of unwanted or unnecessary sounds or phonemes in syllables or words. They are often a result of the child's struggle to speak. Addition of the schwa phoneme *uh* frequently occurs in stuttering. Additions are complication errors seen in motor speech programming disorders. Additions, while also occurring in articulation and phonological disorders, are frequently symptomatic of stuttering, apraxia of speech, and other neuromuscular disorders.

Important aspects of articulation and phonology disorder assessments are **stimulability** testing and **phonological process analyses**. A client who is stimulable can imitate the error phoneme correctly with visual and auditory prompts from the speech-language pathologist. Stimulability assessment can occur in a variety of contexts, including the phoneme in isolation and at the syllable, word, and phrase levels. Phonological process analysis is the assessment and description of the errors, emphasizing their linguistic attributes. **Distinctive feature analysis** involves determining the common linguistic attributes of phonemes that differentiate them from one another, such as place, manner, and voicing. At the conclusion of the diagnostic process, the clinician has a comprehensive picture of the client's articulation and phonology patterns from which to design therapies.

Therapies for Articulation and Phonology Disorders

In the not so distant past, primarily one articulation therapy existed. Certainly, there were variations in the traditional approach based on the client's age and specific factors related to the etiology of the disorder, but essentially the therapy involved **auditory perceptual training**, **production exercises**, and **carryover practice**. Auditory perceptual training consisted of exercises to improve the client's ability to discriminate the error phoneme from others and to learn the perceptual qualities of correctly produced speech. Production exercises began with **simple, noncomplex** articulation of the phoneme and progressed to more **complex, conversational** use of it. The therapy always involved the treatment of only one phoneme until the client had mastered it with greater than 90% success in off-guard, conversational speech (**carryover**). Clinicians first corrected the phoneme that occurred most frequently, and that contributed most to reduction in **intelligibility**, and then addressed phonemes of less importance. Today the traditional approach is best suited for individuals with one or two articulation errors such as a θ/*s* or /*w*/ for /*r*/ substitution, isolated omissions or occasional distortions, and reduced intelligibility.

Plante and Beeson (2004) identify three approaches to articulation therapy for children: **semantic, cross-modality**, and **coarticulatory**. The semantic method emphasizes minimal pairs and changes in meaning that may accompany phonological errors. Cross-modality articulation therapy uses mirrors and other types of feedback to facilitate correct articulatory placement. The coarticulatory approach uses coarticulation and assimilation principles to promote correct articulation. The sounds preceding and following the error are changed to help the child produce correct articulation.

Articulation therapy for structural defects depends on the abnormal structure and often involves concurrent reconstructive surgeries and prosthetics. The type of paralysis or movement disorder seen in neuromuscular impairments also dictates the type of therapy. Therapy for flaccid, spastic, or ataxic paralysis, and for the various movement disorders, has different goals and objectives. Traditional therapies and recent advances in articulation disorders theory have increased the therapy options for clinicians. "The most effective speech-language pathologists working with articulation disorders may be those who are familiar with different approaches and employ the one most appropriate for the individual with the defect. The least effective clinicians, in our opinion, use the same remediation steps for all of their clients" (Plante & Beeson, 2004, p. 83).

Case Studies in Articulation and Phonology Disorders

Case Study 2.1 A Lisp in a 35-Year-Old Professor

OPHELIA BLOCKER

Ophelia Blocker was a unique woman. An "army brat," she was born in Europe, moved to the United States when she was 6 years old, and boasts that she is triracial. Her mother was half Cherokee and half Anglo, and her father is African American. She was intelligent, personable, and firmly committed to military service. She was a captain in the army reserves and recently began teaching two sections of the colloquium courses at a private college. The courses were entitled Valuing Human Diversity in the 21st Century.

Ophelia Blocker also had a discernible lisp that the education system never identified. Perhaps it was because Ophelia moved around so much or because much of her schooling was at army bases, where speech pathology services were often not available. When she became an adult, few people commented on her lisp, and until she started receiving student comments that it was distracting, she considered it unimportant. The dean of the college met with her to discuss the lisp and suggested that she receive articulation therapy at the college's speech and hearing clinic. Ophelia Blocker, never one to avoid sensitive political issues, questioned the labeling of her speech as deviant. She wondered why her speech, which was perfectly intelligible, was considered abnormal instead of just another example of human diversity.

Whether because of her triracial background, her military experiences, or simply the fact that she was intelligent, outspoken, and did not embrace trendy, politically correct beliefs, Ophelia did not accept the idea that she was deviant. She did not adhere to the conventional wisdom that different ways of speaking are necessarily pathological. Ophelia commented to the dean that several faculty members at the college spoke with heavy Korean and Spanish accents and they were not required to undergo therapy, although students complained that they could not understand them. However, the dean insisted that she be evaluated and made it a condition of her continued employment.

During the evaluation, Ophelia's lisp was confirmed. She produced the *th* for the /s/ speech sound. The speech error was consistently present in the initial, medial, and final positions of syllables and words. With careful modeling, Ophelia could produce the /s/ sound with proper tongue placement. Ophelia's oral and facial examination did not show muscle weakness or structural abnormalities. Her teeth were neither missing, jagged, nor jumbled. Oral diadochokinesis was normal, meaning that she could move her tongue rapidly from one position to another. The results of the evaluation showed that Ophelia's lisp was a result of improper learning of tongue placement during /s/ production. The report suggested that because Ophelia had lisped for nearly three decades, her response or habit strength was well established. It would take extensive therapy to eliminate it.

After receiving the evaluation report, Ophelia met with the dean to discuss the required articulation therapy. She maintained her beliefs and challenged the dean about lisping and the concept of diversity. She noted that the college's mission was to embrace diversity and celebrate human individuality. The college was trying to hire a diverse faculty and recruit students from multicultural backgrounds. On the campus, a variety of accents and dialects existed, and those speakers were not required to conform to the Standard American Dialect. Ophelia commented that she was more intelligible than most of the professors with English as a second language.

The dean was also adamant about the negative implications of lisping. He noted that persons are judged by their speech and that "how they talk often speaks louder than what they say." He said that Ophelia should rid herself of the lisp because it would probably be a professional hindrance and reduce her chances of obtaining future employment in higher education. He observed that, rightly or wrongly, most people consider lisping a sign of immature development and reduced intelligence. He suggested that Ophelia watch the movie *My Fair Lady* or see the play *Pygmalion*, on which the movie was based, to see the stereotypes people accept about speech patterns.

Ophelia countered this argument by noting that many past negative stereotypes about people have disappeared. Although progress has been much too slow, she said, many people now accept and even revel in the differences in other people. Ophelia again stated that her speech was intelligible and that negative stereotypes about it were the problems of the people who believed them. She concluded her argument with the statement "I am perfectly content with who I am and how I speak."

The meeting lasted for nearly 2 hours. Ophelia and the dean, both intelligent, articulate, and persuasive debaters, finally reached a conclusion about lisping and diversity. The decision was acceptable to both parties.

Case Study 2.2   A 6-Year-Old Child with a Frontal Lisp

SETH

The speech-language pathologist receives an urgent telephone call from a father requesting a confidential meeting. He wants to discuss his son's speech impediment as soon as possible. The clinician returns the call, and a meeting is scheduled for the end of the week.

The speech-language pathologist identified Seth, the child in question, as having a frontal lisp about 6 months ago during a routine screening. It is caused by Seth's consistent production of the /s/ speech sound as *th*. The frontal lisp occurs in the initial, medial, and final positions of syllables and words. Sometimes articulation disorders occur because the speaker has a shortened lingual frenulum. During the oral-facial examination this structure was found to be normal, and Seth's tongue protrusion, retraction, elevation, and depression were within normal limits for mobility and excursion. The evaluation indicated that Seth *fronted*, meaning that his tongue had anterior placement during /s/ production.

The speech-language pathologist treats many children with /s/ articulation disorders. It is not uncommon for young children to have problems with the /s/ speech sound. About 75% of children acquire normal /s/ speech sound production in all three word positions (initial, medial, final) between the ages of 4 and 5. At 6 years, 8 months, Seth, a second grader, is clearly delayed in acquiring this phoneme.

The therapy Seth receives for the articulation disorder involves the standard sensorimotor approach. First, the clinician trains him to perceive the differences between correct and incorrect productions of the /s/ phoneme. Seth first learns to distinguish the /s/ phoneme from other phonemes when it is spoken by the clinician. Then he learns to distinguish the /s/ phoneme from other fricatives. During the final stages of the auditory perceptual training, Seth learns to distinguish correct from incorrect productions of the /s/ phoneme in the clinician's speech. Finally, he correctly identifies correct and incorrect productions of the /s/ phoneme in his own speech. The clinician uses a game during the auditory perceptual training to make the learning experience enjoyable. Each time Seth makes a correct perceptual judgment, he puts an M&M in a cardboard box. At the end of the therapy sessions, he gets to keep the candy.

During the production phase of the sensorimotor approach, the clinician, using a clinical mirror, shows Seth the proper articulatory placement for the /s/ phoneme. Seth places his tongue in the correct position directly behind his upper incisors. He learns that the tongue should not contact the alveolar ridge but instead provide a "tunnel" for the air to escape. Using the behavior modification principle of shaping, the clinician rewards Seth for successively closer approximations to the correct speech sound production. Each time he produces the /s/ phoneme correctly, the clinician gives him praise and a token. A local bread company has donated to the clinic colorful wrapping tabs used to seal loaves of bread for use as tokens. The tabs can be used to purchase toys, candy, stickers, and games from the clinic's store. Seth has his eye on a remote-controlled pickup truck and works hard in therapy to obtain enough tokens to buy it.

On Friday afternoon, the clinician meets with Seth's father, who explains that he is concerned about his son's sexual orientation. He suspects that he may be gay, given the lisp, and he is worried because Seth does not enjoy the activities popular with other boys of his age. He is deeply concerned and wonders what steps can be taken to reverse his son's apparently developing homosexuality.

Clinical Sidebar 2.2

Lisping in males is sometimes associated with homosexuality. Although this stereotype is sometimes portrayed in films and on television programs, there is no scientific evidence that males who lisp are likely to be homosexual. Do you think this stereotype is common? If so, why do people accept it?

The clinician is surprised at the father's concern and his reaction to Seth's speech disorder but does not dismiss his fear, realizing that a parent's worry is never irrelevant or inappropriate. The clinician simply accepts the father's report as genuine concern for his son and as a product of misinformation and stereotyping. The clinician tells him that lisping is a speech pathology and is not indicative of sexual orientation. In Seth's case, it is a result of misdirecting the airstream during speech production, a common speech disorder in children. The clinician also notes that Seth is making excellent progress in therapy and that his lisp will likely disappear. The father accepts the explanation and seems relieved, but the clinician recommends that he seek counseling to discuss his concerns. There may be larger parenting issues that should be addressed by a family counselor.

Case Study 2.3 An Unintelligible Child with a Phonologically Based Articulation Disorder

CHINA

The teacher was concerned about China's speech development. As a first-year Head Start enrollee, she was completely unintelligible. Although China initiated conversations and responded verbally, all the teacher could discern were strings of unintelligible speech sounds. However, because China was only 3 years old, her speech was not a major concern for the teacher. However, when China enrolled in the second year of the Head Start program and her speech remained unintelligible, the teacher reported it to the speech-language pathologist.

For the teacher, one remarkable aspect of China's communication disorder was that her mother completely understood her jumbled sounds. Once during a parent-teacher conference, China uttered what appeared to be several related sentences that were completely unintelligible to the teacher. When she stopped, her mother matter-of-factly said that she was talking about their family's purchase of a pug puppy. China was describing the pug's unfortunate appearance and saying that they had named it Rosie. Apparently, the mother was able to decipher China's language and had learned her phonological rules.

China was scheduled for a comprehensive articulation and phonological processes assessment. The speech-language pathologist had three goals. First, she wanted to describe China's articulatory and phonological development. The type, form, and consistency of the errors needed to be discovered, in addition to describing their distinctive features. Second, the clinician wanted to decide whether China's speech deviated significantly from that of other children of her age and the effects the disorder had on her functional communication. How consistent were the speech articulation and phonological errors, and what effect did they have on intelligibility? Third, the speech-language pathologist wanted to determine the type of therapy necessary for China's disorder, and to make judgments about the improvement expected with and without therapy.

Phonological testing involved several related but independent subtests. First, a commercially available articulation test was used to inventory China's functional articulation. It identified the phonemes produced incorrectly and the positions of the errors, that is, whether they occurred in the initial, medial, and final positions of words. In addition, China's particular errors were indicated. For each speech sound error discovered on the test, the clinician determined whether it was a distortion, omission, substitution, or addition. The test also had a section to identify the phonological process used by China.

Once the direct phonological testing was completed, the clinician analyzed the features of China's immature and incorrect speech sound production and compared

> **Clinical Sidebar 2.3**
> Intelligibility is the ability to be understood. Although it can be measured by several standardized tests, it is often simply reported as a subjective percentage. For example, the speaker is said to be 20%, 70%, or 100% intelligible. How does rate of speech affect intelligibility? How do you measure rate of speech? At what rate of speech do you become unintelligible?

them with the adult, mature phonological system. This was quickly and accurately done by a commercial computer program. One feature of China's immature phonological system was the substitution of voiceless features by using /t/ and /k/. She would say "Kindy teet ta pug" for "Cindy sees the pug." A significant deterrent to speech intelligibility was China's final consonant deletions—the reduction of consonant-vowel-consonant syllables to consonant-vowel structures—that were apparent in most of the speech sample. For example, China typically said *cu* for *cup*, *tu* for *tub*, and *hou* for *house*. She also engaged in cluster reduction, in which a consonant cluster is reduced to a single consonant, such as when she said *krirrel* for *squirrel*.

Because China's speech disorder was predominantly phonological, the clinician also tested her to determine her overall functional language abilities. She knew that children with significant phonological disorders often also have related language disorders. The test results showed China to have delayed acquisition of receptive vocabulary and grammar, as well as expressive grammatical impairments.

China received daily therapy for the phonology and related language disorders. The goal of therapy was to help her acquire adult-based phonology and consequently improve her speech intelligibility. One successful method was contrast therapy. China was shown pictures of word pairs that differ by one sound. The pictures demonstrated the deficient phonological process. For example, she was shown a series of word pairs with and without final consonant deletion, such as *me–meet* and *car–cart*. China learned not to delete final syllables by attending to the minimal contrasts and the associated phonological processes. Other phonological processes were addressed in a similar manner. China ultimately learned age-appropriate phonology, and her speech became much more intelligible. During "show and tell," China brought Rosie the pug to class and was able to talk at length about her unusual appearance and comical antics.

Case Study 2.4   A /w/ for /r/ Substitution in a Fourth Grader

GERALDO

As an itinerant speech-language pathologist, Wendy enjoys her job and particularly looks forward to Friday afternoons. It is true that at first, Wendy did not want a job that required traveling from one school to another. She thought she wanted to serve only one school, to have one office and one therapy suite, and to interact with the same teachers, support personnel, and administrators. She thought she wanted to see only the children in one school. Nevertheless, after a few weeks on her new job, she was pleasantly surprised to find that being itinerant was a great way to earn a living. On Mondays, Wednesdays, and Fridays, she goes to a small rural school to see her favorite client: a little boy named Geraldo.

What is so enjoyable about her interaction with Geraldo is not that he is improving rapidly, although he is. It is that Geraldo willingly shares his fourth-grade experiences with Wendy. She particularly likes to hear about tall Trudy, who mercilessly teases him. Geraldo freely talks about his confused and mixed feelings about her. This /w/ for /r/

Clinical Sidebar 2.4
Speech-language
pathologists working in
public schools typically
treat more children with
articulation and phonol-
ogy disorders than with
any other type of com-
munication disorder. The
/s/ and /r/ phonemes
are the most common
speech sounds in need
of remediation. Why do
these phonemes pro-
duce the most common
speech sound errors in
school-age children?

substitution brings tears of laughter to Wendy's eyes. Nevertheless, she knows that although a /w/ for /r/ substitution may be appealing in a fourth grader, it is a liability in a teenager or an adult.

Liquid gliding is a common phonological disorder, and some children have several glide substitutions. (*Liquid* is a generic term for the /r/ and /l/ speech sounds). For example, individuals may substitute /r/ for /w/, /l/ for /w/ or other such combinations. When children have more than one liquid gliding substitution, Wendy prefers to treat it as a phonology disorder and to address the errors and the underlying phonological processes. However, as with Geraldo, when only the /w/ for /r/ substitution exists, she prefers to treat it as a functional articulation disorder and uses the traditional therapy that has worked so well historically. There is overlap in the phonological and traditional approaches to /w/ for /r/ substitutions, but Wendy has found that the traditional approach works best when these substitutions occur in isolation.

In this approach, Wendy first addresses Geraldo's auditory perception. She knows that children who substitute one glide for another often do not perceive differences auditorially between the two phonemes. Acoustically, the /w/ is similar to the /r/ phoneme, much more so than it is to the /s/ or /ʤ/ phoneme, for example. Wendy first has Geraldo listen as she says words from a list. Some words have his phoneme, which they have agreed to call the *"r"abbit* sound. As she reads from the word list, Geraldo claps his hands each time he perceives his phoneme. Wendy praises him for his work. Then she has Geraldo perceive the differences between the /r/ phoneme within syllables, telling him to identify it in various positions. After Geraldo has developed this auditory perceptual skill, Wendy teaches him to perceive the /r/ phoneme in words. She reads a list of words with the /r/ phoneme in the initial position, and Geraldo taps the clinical table when the phoneme is detected. Once he has mastered this auditory perception, Wendy has him do similar activities with words having the /r/ in the final and medial positions. She also has Geraldo play games in which he distinguishes the /w/ from the /r/ sound.

After the auditory perceptual exercises, Wendy begins the production phase of the traditional articulation therapy for Geraldo's /w/ for /r/ substitution. During the evaluation, stimulability testing found that Geraldo is unable to produce the correct /r/ phoneme by imitation. In addition, Wendy conducts deep testing, in which the phonetic contexts of his misarticulation are altered and the circumstances that resulted in correct production discovered. By varying the phonemes that precede and follow the /r/, Wendy is able to get Geraldo to produce a correct /r/ speech sound in isolation. Geraldo is able to produce a correct /r/ in the word combination *fun–run*. Eventually, Geraldo can consistently produce the /r/ sound in isolation, and Wendy rewards him for each correct production.

As Wendy continues with the production phase, Geraldo is taught to produce the /r/ phoneme in more complex contexts. First, he produces the speech sound in the initial position of syllables such as *ra*, *ree*, and *roo*. Then he produces the phoneme in the final position of syllables such as *eer*, *oor*, and *ahr*. Finally, during syllable production, Geraldo learns to produce the /r/ phoneme in syllable contexts where his phoneme is in the middle.

Now that Geraldo has mastered correct production of the /r/ phoneme in isolation and in syllables, Wendy moves to the next level of articulatory complexity: words. Similar to the production exercises for syllables, Geraldo first works on producing the /r/ phoneme in the initial position. Wendy shows him photo cards and word lists, and he is soon able to produce it. Then he works on the /r/ in the final and medial positions of words. Soon he is producing it correctly in all three positions of words.

Continuing to increase the articulatory complexity, Wendy has Geraldo create sentences and phrases using words with the /r/ phoneme. First, she encourages him to attend carefully to the /r/ sound production. As his mastery increases, she gradually creates conversations in which Geraldo attends less and less to the /r/ sound production. The goal is to gradually help Geraldo learn to use the /r/ phoneme correctly in off-guard speech. Wendy also enlists the help of his teachers and parents to cue him to use the phoneme correctly in the classroom and at home. Soon Geraldo has mastered the correct production of the /r/ phoneme in all contexts and has carried over what he learned in individual therapy to all aspects of his life.

Case Study 2.5   Group Therapy for Articulation and Phonology Disorders

NICOLE, YONKEL, TARA, AND JAMES ROBERT

Circle is their favorite activity in group therapy. In circle, Nicole, Yonkel, Tara, and James Robert get to stand together in the small therapy suite, hold hands, and play enjoyable games. As first graders, they are not certain why they spend time together in circle or why they leave the regular classroom 3 days a week. All they know is that circle is fun, and as they settle down for therapy, they coax the speech teacher to begin. On Mondays, Wednesdays, and Fridays, at precisely 10:15 a.m., the teachers and students can hear the chant "Circle, circle, circle" resonate through the halls of the small elementary school.

Because the clinician believes that two or more brief therapy sessions are more beneficial than one long session, the children are seen in group therapy for 10 to 15 minutes twice daily. The frequent, short sessions are more important for younger children because their memory and attention are limited. Consequently, Nicole, Yonkel, Tara, and James Robert have circle in the morning and afternoon three times per week.

Nicole, Yonkel, Tara, and James Robert particularly look forward to this week's group activities with their speech teacher. They are excited because next week is Christmas break and celebration of all of the winter holidays. The speech teacher has decorated the therapy room with pictures of snowy sleigh rides, festive family feasts, menorah operas, reindeer, frosty snowmen, and sleds shooting down crisp winter

Clinical Sidebar 2.5
In articulation and
phonology therapy,
speech-language pathol-
ogists use theme
pictures and words. The
themes usually focus on
topics discussed in the
children's classroom,
including their neighbor-
hoods, family members,
birthdays, and vacations.
Why do speech-
language pathologists
integrate their therapies
into classroom activities?

urban hills. Because the children are working on the /k/ and /g/ phonemes, the winter holiday themes focus on those sounds.

During circle, the children discuss the pictures on the wall. Nicole happily describes a picture of red-cheeked children riding in a sleigh being pulled through the snow by a high-stepping white horse. Yonkel describes the menorah, the significance of eight candles, and the miracle of oil lasting for 8 days. In cele-bration of Chanukah, he talks about potato pancakes, chocolate money, and the game in which children spin a four-sided top. Tara recalls her family's Thanksgiving dinner, including all of the fixings—a huge turkey, dressing, potatoes, salads, and pumpkin pies—and Tara recalls her grandparents traveling from Iowa for the dinner. James Robert, or "Jim Bob" as his family calls him, talks at length about a mechanical toy Santa will doubtless bring him. As the children talk, the speech-language pathologist cues them to pay particular attention to the /k/ and /g/ words. After everyone has had an opportunity to talk in circle, the therapist has them say the following words: *Yonkel, candles, Chanukah, pancakes, Thanksgiv-ing, Christmas, turkey, cheek, pumpkins, gold, chocolate, game, dressing.* The speech sounds are made correctly by all of the children.

After circle, the children read the special story prepared by the speech-language pathologist. A computer program structures the story and the colorful illustrations. The story involves a magical snowman built by boys and girls after the first snowfall. To add interest for the speech students, the clinician has included the names Nicole, Yonkel, Tara, and James Robert in the story; it is as if they had created Frosty on that cold winter's day. The therapist reads the story and the children describe the pictures, using /k/ and /g/ phonemes appropriately and accurately.

The clinician has created a "speech club" with all of the children as members. To exit the session and return to the classroom, each child must whisper a passage of secret words to the speech-language pathologist. Of course, the words must be articulated properly or the teacher will not open the door. Each child correctly whis-pers the passage and returns to the classroom. To protect the secrecy of the group, the passage cannot be divulged; however, it is rumored that it contains several words with the /k/ and /g/ phonemes.

Case Study 2.6 Augmentative and Alternative Communication Devices for Two Children with Oral-Facial Paralysis

JUANITA AND DECON

For Jodie, seeing only preschoolers is just fine. In fact, she prefers to work with very young children, having spent nearly two decades working in a hospital as a speech-language pathologist. In the hospital setting, she worked primarily with adults, often geriatric patients. Jodie found the work challenging, exciting, and, much too often, very stressful. In the medical setting, she spent most of her workday helping people with strokes, progressive neurological diseases, brain tumors, and traumatic brain injuries. She finally decided that she needed a change, and when the position in the public school opened, she was hired almost immediately. Now Jodie's oldest client is 6 years old, and she spends her workday with young children who have bright futures.

Jodie's new job is not free from stress, nor are the challenges her clients face less profound. She has the usual scheduling problems and occasional professional differences. She has two preschoolers, Juanita and Decon, with major paralytic speech disorders. Their oral-facial paralysis is so severe that both require augmentative and alternative communication devices. The decision to have them use these devices was not easy. Jodie would have preferred to have them develop their existing neuromotor abilities, compensate for their deficiencies, and eventually learn to talk without assistance. However, in both children, the oral-facial paralysis is too severe; they are not likely to ever communicate meaningfully without the use of these devices. This is not to say that oral-motor exercise and speech precision therapies are absent from their IEPs. It simply means that the technological marvels are now part of their communication repertory.

Juanita was born with tongue paralysis; the doctors do not know what caused it. Apparently her hypoglossal cranial nerve was injured before or during birth. The hypoglossal nerve, or cranial nerve XII as it is technically called, is primarily a motor nerve and supplies the nerve impulses to the intrinsic muscles of the tongue. The neurologist speculates that the upper cervical vertebrae were dislocated during delivery, causing the lower motor neuron damage and flaccid musculature.

Several years have been devoted to strengthening Juanita's flaccid tongue muscles, with little improvement. Exercises include protruding and lateralizing the tongue with resistance and pushing it against the alveolar ridge and cheek. Speech drills are used to improve oral diadochokinesis, rapid tongue movements, and repeatedly producing phonemes such as /d/ and /t/. However, the improvement has been marginal and Juanita has become increasingly frustrated at her inability to speak intelligibly. When introduced to the new communication device, she took to it with enthusiasm.

Because Juanita has no limb paralysis, she can use the direct select device, in which she touches words and icons and the computer speaks for her. This particular device also remembers frequently used phrases and can generate variations of new ones. Jodie has her use it in conjunction with oral speech, and Juanita is now able to communicate with her peers and teachers. Technology and oral-facial therapies have helped bridge the communication gap for Juanita and are creating new types of socialization for her.

Decon, the other child with dysarthria, has spastic paraplegia and spends most of his time in a wheelchair. Decon suffered from lack of oxygen to his brain due to reduction of the blood supply before or during birth. This caused severe spastic dysarthria, rendering him nearly mute. As with Juanita, Decon's intelligence is largely unaffected by the neurological damage. Because of the bilateral upper motor neuron damage, Decon has spastic dysarthria and severe motor impairments throughout his body. He is almost incapable of producing meaningful speech sounds and has suffered from swallowing problems throughout life. His other physical limitations are as severe as his speech disorders, requiring extensive physical and occupational therapy.

Because Decon uses a wheelchair, the augmentative and alternative communication device is mounted on it. There is also a desk mount for the times when Decon prefers to sit in a classroom with the other children. For his wheelchair, a special folding mount is required because Decon rides a bus to and from school. Though the bus has wheelchair accommodation, a special setup is necessary so that the device is not damaged during the ride and when loading and unloading.

Because of his paralysis, Decon requires two sensor switches. The first switch is ultrathin and easily fits into his spastic hand. A red light appears when the power is on, and a blue one flashes when he activates the communication device. Thanks to a grant from a parent association affiliated with the school, Decon can also use a new fiberoptic eye-blink switch. Purposeful eye blinks adjust the scanning of the communication board, and the device can distinguish between random eye blinks and purposeful ones. Decon wears a head strap that has a reflective device for interpreting eye blinks.

Jodie has spent a lot of time learning to use the augmentative and alternative communication devices. In therapy, she shows the children how to refine and expand their use. They play games, learn cooperative activities, give directions, and engage in turn-taking. Jodie also drills them on speech sound production, hoping that someday they may be able to learn to make intelligible speech sounds and not have to use augmentative and alternative communication devices.

SUMMARY

Articulation and phonology disorders disrupt or eliminate the ability to form speech sounds and produce articulate speech. It takes several years for children to master articulation and to learn the phonological rules of language, and for some, articulation and phonology therapies are required. There are several causative factors in articulation and phonology disorders including language delay, structural anomalies, neuromuscular disorders, emotional precipitants, and hearing loss. Diagnosis involves describing these disorders in all contexts so that appropriate therapies may be conducted. For some individuals with severe articulation and phonology disorders, augmentative and alternative communication devices may be required.

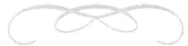

Study and Discussion Questions

1. List and describe the primary fixed, mobile, hard, and soft articulators.

2. Transcribe your name phonetically.

3. What factors must you consider when determining whether a child has articulation and phonology delay?

4. Describe the difference between nonstandard and substandard speech production.

5. List and briefly discuss the structural abnormalities that can affect articulation.

6. Compare and contrast apraxia of speech and the dysarthria's effect on articulation.

7. What are some indications that a child has an emotionally based articulation disorder? What types of referrals are appropriate for this type of communication disorder?

8. Compute your chronological age in years, months, and days.

9. Describe the three-by-three system of diagnosing articulation disorders.

10. Compare and contrast the traditional articulation therapy and those described by Plante and Beeson (2004).

Recommended Reading and Film

Alvarez, L., & Kolker, A. (1987). *American tongues* [Film]. New York: Center for New American Media.

   This film provides an excellent overview of accent and dialect in the United States.

Culbertson, W., & Tanner, D. (2001). Clinical comparisons: Phonological processes and their relationship to traditional phoneme norms. *Infant-Toddler Intervention, 11*(1), 15–25.

   This article compares and contrasts phonological processes and traditional phoneme norms showing a strong relationship in extinction and acquisition age levels.

Plante, E., & Beeson, P. (2004). *Communication and communication disorders: A clinical introduction* (2nd ed.). Boston: Allyn & Bacon.

   This introductory book has an excellent chapter on articulation and phonology disorders.

Tanner, D. (2003). *Exploring communication disorders: A 21st century introduction through literature and media.* Boston: Allyn & Bacon.

This introductory book has a chapter on articulation and phonology disorders and several examples of how they are portrayed in literature and the media.

Wise, R. J. S., Greene, J., Büchel, C., & Scott, S. K. (1999). Brain regions involved in articulation. *Lancet, 353,* 1057–1061.

This research article, published in a respected journal, examines the brain regions associated with the articulatory plan.

CHAPTER THREE

Stuttering

There is no such thing as conversation. It is an illusion. There are intersecting monologues. That is all.

Rebecca West

Chapter Preview: In this chapter, the fluency disorder of stuttering is defined and discussed. Theories about the etiology of stuttering and diagnostic issues are presented. Treatment of the visible features of stuttering, auditory symptoms, anxiety, and associated negative emotions, as well as the influence of the disorder on self-concept and speech-related self-esteem, are also reviewed. Case studies include a precocious 3-year-old whose mental abilities exceed her speech motor skills, a mentally impaired–mentally retarded person who stutters, and a 5-year-old boy in whom stuttering was prevented. Other case studies illustrate various treatment approaches and an account of therapy in a camp situation.

OVERVIEW OF STUTTERING

Stuttering is a **fluency** disorder affecting the ability to make speech sounds effortlessly. Fluency is the smoothness and ease with which units of speech are combined in oral language. A fluency disorder is an impairment in the ability to produce speech without interjections, fillers, blocks, or hesitations. Stuttering is an age-old communication disorder, and it occurs in all cultures and languages. The ancient Greeks referred to stuttering, and some religious scholars believe that Moses stuttered. Public figures, celebrities, and entertainers with a stuttering problem include Charles Darwin, King George VI, Winston Churchill, George Burns, Marilyn Monroe, Bob Newhart, James Earl Jones, and Bruce Willis. Most stuttering begins in childhood but can also occur in adults. The incidence and prevalence of stuttering vary among cultures; generally in the United States, about 1% of the population stutters. Studies on the incidence and prevalence of stuttering are difficult to compare and analyze because there are many definitions of stuttering, the disorder usually develops gradually, and individuals are never perfectly fluent all the time.

Definition of Stuttering

Speech fluency occurs on a continuum; a range of **normal dysfluencies** appears in human speech patterns, and there is no clear line separating normally fluent speech from stuttering.

When talking, all persons repeat sounds, syllables, words, and phrases. They also hesitate and pause during speech, particularly when distracted, when thinking about the topic, or when selecting the appropriate word to use. Sometimes persons prolong sounds during speech and interject words and sounds such as *you know* and *uh*. These **repetitions, prolongations**, and **hesitations** are usually produced subconsciously and are typical speech patterns occurring in all persons. However, some persons display these behaviors more frequently and with more severity, and they consider themselves stutterers. Stuttering and **cluttering**, a **verbal thought-organization** disorder, are the two major fluency-disrupting speech pathologies. In cluttering, the speaker is usually unaware of the dysfluencies, speaks rapidly, and has a brief attention span and poor concentration. Because speech-language pathologists rarely treat cluttering as a clinical entity, this chapter addresses the diagnosis and treatment of stuttering.

There are many definitions of stuttering, but Van Riper's (1973, 1992) has the most clinical use. He defines stuttering as a word improperly patterned in time and the speaker's reaction thereto. According to Van Riper, a person who stutters has an abnormal number of dysfluencies and reacts negatively to them. Words are improperly patterned in time by repetitions, prolongations, and blocks in the flow of speech, and the **negative emotions** may include anxiety, fear, embarrassment, and guilt. Persons with stuttering may also use certain behaviors to avoid or escape from the moment of stuttering. These can take the form of avoiding eye contact, closing the eyes, slapping the hand, jerking the head, and others. Following is a comprehensive definition of a person who stutters. It serves as the basis for the discussion of this communication disorder.

> An individual who improperly patterns phonemes, syllables, words and/or phrases in time; who experiences classically-conditioned negative emotional reactions to disfluent speech and associated stimuli and who may engage in visible avoidance and escape behaviors when confronted with disfluent speech or associated stimuli. *(Tanner, Belliveau, & Siebert, 1995, p. 6)*

Etiology of Stuttering: Nature or Nurture?

The etiology of stuttering has been debated for decades, and one question consistently arises: Is stuttering caused by learning and environmental factors or is it a result of physical, organic irregularities? Over the years, organic, learning, and psychological theories have been advanced to explain the etiology of stuttering. At the core of this debate is the age-old question asked about many human maladies: Is stuttering caused by nature or nurture? Currently, many speech scientists and clinicians believe that the organic theories explain why some persons develop stuttering.

Organic Theories of Stuttering

According to the **organic theories** of stuttering, some persons are **predisposed** to stuttering because of neurological or physical anomalies. They have brain damage or irregularities, neurological impairments, or muscular deficits that impair speech fluency. Also, some authorities believe that stuttering is caused by a problem with auditory feedback when the person speaks. There is also mounting evidence of a gene for stuttering. According to Owens, Metz, and Haas (2000), 50% of persons who stutter have a relative who stuttered. This high rate of stuttering within families may support a genetic link to the disorder or it may simply suggest similar child-rearing practices among generations of these families. Most authorities on stuttering acknowledge that if there is a gene for stuttering, it **predisposes** the person to stutter and that environmental factors play a role in **precipitating** and **perpetuating** the disorder. There are several other organic theories of stuttering linking the disorder to brain abnormalities and neurological impairments. New brain scanning technologies, such as positron emission tomography (PET), have provided evidence of a neurological basis for stuttering (Kroll & DeNil, 1998). However, with regard to the organic theories of stuttering, it should be noted that even if stuttering is a physically based disorder, currently there are no surgeries or medications to eliminate it; therapeutic prevention and management are required.

Psychological Theories of Stuttering

The **psychological theories** focus on two aspects of stuttering. First, some theories propose that stuttering is directly caused by psychological catalysts. These range from repressed needs, to conflicts between the id and superego, to unspeakable feelings and conversion reactions such as oral fixations and repressed hostility. The purely psychological etiology of stuttering has been generally discounted, except for those persons with late onset of the disorder. When stuttering begins in adults, it is likely to be hysterically based and a result of psychological trauma. The most frequent psychiatric problems observed in psychogenic stuttering include conversion reactions, anxiety, and hysterical neurosis (Duffy & Baumgartner, 1997). Van Riper (1973, 1992) believes that late-onset hysterical stuttering is fundamentally different from childhood stuttering.

The second aspect of the psychological theories involves the role of stuttering in shaping personality. This too is a controversial aspect of stuttering. Does stuttering affect a person psychologically? Is there a **stuttering personality**? Decades of research on this subject have not provided a clear consensus, but it is logical that stuttering, like many disabilities, affects a person's social interactions, self-concept, and interpersonal relationships. Crichton-Smith (2002) found that stuttering can have a limiting effect on the individual's life, especially in the areas of employment, education, and self-esteem. However, few studies have shown that stuttering causes the person to be dramatically affected psychologically. Most persons who stutter report anxiety and embarrassment while speaking, and dealing with frequent trepidation and other negative emotions creates psychological challenges. Of course, not all persons who stutter have anxiety while stuttering, and they also have the anxiety-free normal nonfluencies seen in nonstutterers. Stuttering can be troublesome, but it is not psychologically and socially devastating to most individuals. However, rarely is psychotherapy alone able to cure or significantly decrease stuttering.

Learning Theories of Stuttering

The two **primary learning theories** of stuttering, summarized below, propose that the disorder is the result of (a) the **reinforcement** and subsequent increase in the number of normal nonfluencies or (b) the disruptive effects of **negative emotional learning** on speech fluency. Both learning theories suggest the etiology of the disorder and provide for therapeutic intervention.

The **operant conditioning theory** suggests that persons develop stuttering because the normal nonfluencies that everyone displays are rewarded and thus increase in frequency and duration. Children, particularly between the ages of 3 and 7 years, display frequent normal nonfluencies during speech, especially when excited. **Environmental rewards** are present for the nonfluencies, thus increasing the likelihood of their recurrence. Environmental rewards for the child include attention from parents and teachers, noninterruption, special status among peers, and other individually dependent factors. The more dysfluencies the child displays, the more frequent are the rewards for the behavior. Over time, the dysfluencies are shaped into unique patterns of stuttering. The treatment approaches for these operantly conditioned behaviors consist of removing rewards for stuttering and rewarding normally fluent speech patterns.

The **classical conditioning theory** suggests that stuttering is the result of disruptive effects of **anxiety** during speech (Brutten & Shoemaker, 1967). According to this theory, anxiety disrupts the fine motor functioning of speech muscles and causes dysfluencies. Because of **classical** (Pavlovian) **conditioning**, the individual experiences anxiety in connection with certain sounds, words, situations, and persons. The anxiety is generated from within because of **verbal impotence** and from the audience because of ridicule. Both external and internal sources of anxiety are paired with the stuttering stimuli, and a **vicious cycle** of stuttering and anxiety is set in motion. According to the classical conditioning theory, the therapy for stuttering consists of **systematic desensitization** in much the same way that other anxiety-based disorders are treated.

The above learning theories of stuttering have two major differences in their assumptions about the disorder. First, they differ on the nature of the dysfluencies. The operant theory considers the dysfluencies to be excessive normal disruptions of speech output. The classical theory believes them to be abnormal dysfluencies resulting from the disruptive effects of anxiety and other negative emotions. Second, while classical models of stuttering acknowledge the effects of reinforcement on behavior, they focus primarily on stimuli—the factors that prompt stuttering. Conversely, while operant models acknowledge stuttering stimuli, they focus primarily on effects—the rewards and punishments for episodes of stuttering.

Multiple Causation Theory of Stuttering

Since no single theory about the etiology of stuttering has been accepted after nearly a century of research, it is likely to have **multiple causation**. Some persons may develop stuttering because of a **psychological shock** or **trauma**. For example, soldiers in combat sometimes develop stuttering because of extreme stress. Other persons may have learned to stutter. For them, it is a **self-perpetuating** bad habit that is difficult to break. There is probably a **genetic basis** to stuttering, and some children may be born with a predisposition to this disorder. In many patients, genetics, learning, and psychological problems may work together to cause stuttering. Stuttering is a complex communication disorder, and so is the search for its cause or causes.

Diagnosing Stuttering in Children

Bloodstein (1995) reports that about 5% of the population have stuttered at some point in their lives. Many more children than adults go through periods of excessive dysfluencies but do not consider themselves to have a stutter. Parents frequently become concerned that their children may be developing a stutter. For these reasons, speech-language pathologists, particularly those working in educational settings, often must screen and evaluate large numbers of children to see whether their dysfluencies are normal or if they are developing a stutter. Diagnosing stuttering in children is a complex, important, and necessary professional responsibility and is part of the scope of practice for all speech-language pathologists.

Although no clinician wants to make diagnostic mistakes, two types of errors can be made when diagnosing stuttering in children. First, a clinician can make a **false-positive** diagnosis and decide that a child is stuttering when, in fact, this is not so. The child may be going through a period of excessive dysfluencies, and his or her parents and teachers may be concerned about them. However, in reality, the dysfluencies, though excessive, are normal and temporary. Eventually, the child will outgrow them and display normal nonfluencies typical of all speakers. The second type of mistake is the **false-negative** diagnosis in which the clinician believes that the child is normally nonfluent and will eventually outgrow the excessive dysfluencies. In reality, the child is stuttering.

Clinicians want to make correct diagnoses at all times, but sometimes errors occur. In diagnosing stuttering in children, the false-positive error is more detrimental than the false-negative one. Clinicians should attempt to be error-free, but if an error is made, it is better to make a false-negative diagnosis than to diagnose a normally fluent child as one who is stuttering. The reasoning behind this principle is discussed below.

As noted above, a false-negative diagnosis suggests that the child is not stuttering when, in fact, he or she is. Consequently, a child who needs therapy does not receive it. The negative effects of this error include lost treatment time, and the stuttering is likely to get worse. However, eventually the abnormal dysfluencies will be correctly evaluated and the child placed in therapy. Sometimes a false-positive diagnosis is more detrimental than a false-negative one. A normally fluent child with excessive repetitions, prolongations, and hesitations may be regularly pulled from the classroom and taken to speech therapy. As a result, he or she may become unduly self-conscious about speech fluency, which can contribute to the development of stuttering. The theory that misdiagnosis can contribute to stuttering development is a long-standing clinical concept known as the **diagnosogenic theory of stuttering** (Johnson, 1938).

The frequency and types of dysfluencies displayed by the child can indicate whether he or she is normally nonfluent or stuttering. A diagnostic gray area is called **incipient** or

Table 3.1 Indicators of Stuttering in Children

Struggle	Forced production of sounds, syllables, and words
Schwa vowel	Production of the vowel *uh* between or within words
Tremor	Rapid, repetitive movements of the lips, tongue, or jaw
Number and duration of the dysfluencies	More than two repetitions per word; lengthy prolongations and blocks
Circumlocutions	Using substitute words for ones that are feared or cannot be spoken
Eye contact	Little or no eye contact during conversations to avoid negative reactions of listeners
Pauses	Silent gaps between and, more significantly, within words
Avoidance	Postponement or refusal to talk due to the negativity associated with dysfluent speech
Pitch	Pitch rises as a consequence of increased laryngeal tension during speech
Frustration	Anger or crying as manifestations of inability to speak easily
Airflow	Gasping at the end of an utterance

developmental stuttering because it may not be clear that a particular child is or is not stuttering. Table 3.1 shows some speech and ancillary behaviors that separate normally nonfluent children from those who may be stuttering (Tanner, 1990). Struggle with speech, airflow disruptions within words, and the excessive use of the **schwa vowel**, *uh*, are important signs of stuttering. Unfortunately, because of the wide variety of symptoms, there are no reliable and valid diagnostic tests that can be administered to show definitively which children are stuttering and which ones are normally nonfluent. Diagnosing stuttering in children is an ongoing clinical judgment based on observations, test scores, parental interviews, and direct assessment.

Treatment of Stuttering

Several methods of evaluating and treating stuttering exist. Some clinicians separate stuttering into **core** and **accessory** features. The core features are the repetitions, prolongations, and blocks in speech, and the accessory or secondary features are eye squints, hand slaps, head jerks, and the like. Other clinicians evaluate and treat **overt** and **covert** symptoms of the disorder. The overt symptoms are the disruptions in speech fluency, and the covert features are the anxiety reactions, embarrassment, shame, and guilt that many persons experience while stuttering. In children, **true stuttering** is often differentiated from normal nonfluencies and incipient stuttering. One way of evaluating and treating stuttering is to separate the symptoms of the disorder into (a) **what is heard**; (b) **what is seen**; (c) **what is felt** by the person before, during, and after the moment of stuttering; and (d) the **effects of the disorder on the person's personality** (Tanner, 1994, 1999b, 2003c; Tanner et al., 1995). Each of these symptoms provides a framework for evaluation and treatment of this complex communication disorder.

Stuttering: What Is Heard

The **audible** symptoms of stuttering are repetitions, prolongations, and blocks. Repetitions occur on sounds, syllables, and words. For example, a stuttering person may say, "s, s, s, Susan" or "Please pass the coff, coff, coff" or "I want, want, want." Repetitions can also occur on phrases, for example, "I want to, I want to, I want to go outside." Prolongation is the "stretching out" of certain speech sounds, usually continuants. For example, the word *soup* might be said as *sssssssssssoup*. Blocks are silent gaps or pauses between or within words, such as "May I [pause] have some pop [pause] corn?" Many persons who stutter have a combination of repetitions, prolongations, and blocks.

There are several techniques for managing the audible symptoms of stuttering. The **fluent stuttering** approach and the **Van Riper approach** are widely used. The goal of fluent stuttering is to have the person who stutters do so less abnormally. Early in the treatment of stuttering, it was found that if persons who stutter are admonished for the behavior and attempt *not* to stutter, often the result is an increase in the frequency and severity of the disorder. In fluent stuttering therapy, the person is permitted to stutter but is taught to do so **unobtrusively**. According to Hegde (2001), Van Riper's approach is "[a]n extensive, early, and influential treatment program for stuttering; also described as stuttering modification therapy; [the] goal is to teach less abnormal, socially more acceptable stuttering, not necessarily normal fluency" (p. 487). When persons who stutter become proficient in this technique, many can modify their stuttering to the extent that the audience is unaware of the audible symptoms of stuttering.

Stuttering: What Is Seen

The **visible features** of stuttering are highly individualized **avoidance** and **escape** behaviors. They are used by the person who stutters to avoid the moment of stuttering or to escape from it once it occurs. As noted above, they can include head jerks, inappropriate eye blinks, lack of eye contact, hand slaps, inappropriate articulatory gestures, biting the lips, turning the head, twisting the trunk, and others. Many of these behaviors are learned over time and become integral parts of the stuttering pattern. In many persons who stutter, as the stutter increases in severity, they activate more avoidance and escape behaviors. These behaviors also reflect the order in which they were learned; the first-learned behaviors are activated first, the second-learned ones are activated next, and so forth.

The visible features of stuttering can be modified through **behavior modification**. In adults, often it is only necessary to bring negative visible behaviors to their attention. This can be done by videotaping speech segments or by having them observe their face and upper body in a mirror while talking. Adults will usually eliminate head jerks, eye blinks, hand slaps, inappropriate articulatory gestures, lip biting, and head turning, and will maintain eye contact with regular encouragement and direction from the clinician. Children often require a system of rewards in which normal facial expressions are rewarded and abnormal visible features discouraged. It is often desirable to reward normal facial expressions and body movements rather than to discourage abnormal ones. When dealing with the visible features of stuttering, it is not necessary to address the audible symptoms; only the aberrant facial and body aspects of stuttering are targeted for elimination.

Stuttering: Anxiety and Associated Negative Emotions

Most therapies recognize the role **anxiety and associated negative emotions** play in precipitating and perpetuating the stuttering moment. While not all persons who stutter experience negative emotions during stuttering, most report that it is unpleasant and anxiety-provoking. Individuals who stutter also have the anxiety-free, normal nonfluencies experienced by all speakers. However, a comprehensive stuttering program must address the client's anxieties and negative emotions that are associated with dysfluent speech.

Brutten and Shoemaker (1967) first proposed that stuttering could be treated by eliminating anxiety and the negative emotions associated with speaking. Although simply removing anxiety and negative emotions may not be sufficient to cure or significantly reduce stuttering, the affective aspects of the disorder must be addressed. Stuttering can be prompted by past associations with certain **sounds**, **words**, **situations**, and **persons**, and desensitization to them can eliminate them as cues.

The process of **systematically desensitizing** a person to stuttering begins with the client identifying stimuli or cues that prompt the disorder. Several sessions are usually necessary to identify the specific sounds, words, situations, and persons that cause anxiety and associated negative emotions during speech. They are listed in descending order of importance—the most important stimuli first, followed by the second, third, and so forth.

Once the client has listed the stuttering stimuli, **relaxation training** begins. This training has two goals. First, it teaches the client how to relax the body and create a neutral or positive emotional state that can be used in desensitizing. Second, it teaches the client to reduce **hypertense** speech musculature. In many clients, stuttering and struggling with speech are synonymous, and reducing hypertense speech musculature during speaking can produce an immediate improvement in speech fluency. A taped sequence involving **progressive relaxation**, **meditation**, and **autosuggestion** can be used to increase the client's ability to obtain the necessary relaxation and the neutral or positive emotions for desensitization (Tanner, 1991).

Once the client is trained in progressive relaxation, **stuttering stimuli** are paired during states of positive or neutral emotions. The client uses the sounds, words, or phrases repeatedly while experiencing these emotions. He or she also practices using **anxiety-provoking** sounds, words, and phrases in stressful situations and talking to persons from the stuttering hierarchy list. When it is not practical to talk to persons or speak in stuttering-provoking situations, such as talking to a police officer or a large audience, vicarious de-conditioning is employed; role playing and imagery can be used. Group stuttering therapy is also a way of deconditioning clients to stuttering stimuli.

Stuttering and Its Effects on Personality

The effect of stuttering on personality is a controversial topic. Some authorities believe that a **stuttering personality** exists. They assume that stuttering affects all persons in similar ways and invariably alters the way they view and interact with the world. However, Bloodstein (1981), after an extensive review of the literature, suggests that there is no absolute stuttering personality or even definable personality traits of persons who stutter. As a group, persons who stutter are diverse, and they vary greatly with regard to the severity of the disorder and their reactions to it. However, a person who developed stuttering as a young child and suffered years of **ridicule** and **rejection** because of the disorder may have an altered self-concept and reduced self-esteem, particularly in regard to speech-related activities. As Rolin (2000, p. 106) suggests, "As we consider the molding of self-image in the stuttering individual, we are clear that we refer not to a unique 'stuttering personality' but to a special way in which the person perceives him- or herself." Rejection and ridicule, particularly for the child, can create special self-concept and self-esteem challenges. A creative 9-year-old boy put his feelings about stuttering and rejection in a song (Tanner & Lafferty, 2001):

People Say Stupid Things
Garrison Fawcett

People say stupid things,
I know why but they stink,
Makes me sad,
When they're bad,
I wish they would,
Be nice to me,
I wish they would,
Just go away,
Then I would have a better day

Chorus: Na na na na na

This is why people say,
Stupid things,
When they're mad,
They say stupid things. (p. 31)

Guitar (1998) considers the person's feeling about stuttering to be as much a part of the disorder as the actual dysfluencies. Linn and Caruso (1998) suggest that stuttering in adults is a major obstacle to finding a life partner. Many counseling approaches are available to help clients explore, evaluate, and analyze social issues related to stuttering. Group therapy, stuttering camps, and support organizations provide valuable interaction with other persons who stutter and address self-concept and self-esteem concerns. Referral to a psychologist or counselor is appropriate for some persons whose stuttering is a major deterrent to **self-actualization**, employment, or the development and maintenance of relationships. Speech-language pathologists address speech-related self-esteem and self-concept development in children by making speaking a rewarding and enjoyable experience. The child's parents are also involved in achieving these objectives.

Case Studies in Stuttering

Case Study 3.1   A 3-Year-Old Child with Confirmed Stuttering

ALICE LA CLAIRE

Michelle La Claire calls the speech and hearing clinic, anxiously reporting that her 3-year-old daughter, Alice, may be starting to stutter. The clinician listens as the worried mother describes her daughter's speech and language development and her suspected stuttering problem. An appointment is scheduled, and after the call ends, the clinician mentions the upcoming evaluation to a colleague. She agrees that a severe and established stuttering problem at 3 years of age is implausible but not impossible. Without making judgments about the veracity of the mother's report, they acknowledge that the evaluation will be interesting and that careful, detailed testing will be necessary.

Clinical Sidebar 3.1
Stuttering can be prevented in the majority of children if it is caught early. Preventing stuttering is more successful than trying to cure it. The longer a person has stuttered, the stronger the habit and the response, making it more difficult to modify or eliminate. Why else is stuttering easier to prevent than to cure?

The speech and hearing clinic is the only private provider of services for persons with communication disorders in the small city. The clinic sees few children who stutter because these services are covered by the public schools. Two speech-language pathologists and an audiologist serve walk-ins who come to the clinic, and Michelle and Alice arrive promptly at 9:00 a.m. The receptionist takes the necessary background and payment information, and at 9:15 the stuttering evaluation commences. One clinician begins interviewing Michelle in her office, while the other plays with Alice on the floor of the "Kid's Room" of the clinic. This large room is cluttered with hundreds of toys and games, a child's kitchen consisting of toy plates and utensils, and an oven using the heat from a light bulb for baking. There is even a 5-foot-tall playhouse made of rubber walls and plastic windows, with a door allowing only children to enter.

To say that Alice is precocious is an understatement. She has just turned 3, and the clinician evaluating her is amazed at her speech and language development. Talking to Alice is like talking to a small adult. The first statement Alice makes is, "What a beautiful playhouse; may I go inside?" Unfortunately, the statement is made with a stutter. She actually says, "Wh, wh, wh, wh, what a beaut, beautiful pppppppplayhouse. [pause] Mmmmmay I g, g, g, go inssssssssside?"

The clinician interviewing Michelle asks about Alice's delivery, when she first sat up, crawled, walked, and talked, and other questions about her growth and maturation. Every maturational and growth milestone shows Alice to be an extremely bright youngster. The clinician also queries Michelle about relatives with a stuttering problem and is not surprised to learn that Alice's uncle stutters. In college, the clinician learned that stuttering runs in families. She also asks how much time Alice spends with the stuttering relative. Apparently, this is a close-knit family, and Alice's frequent babysitters are her aunt and her stuttering uncle. The clinician also asks Michelle to describe stuttering because sometimes parents consider normal nonfluencies to be abnormal.

The clinician evaluating Alice is awestruck at the child's advanced language structure and dumbfounded by her stuttering. As Alice talks about the steps necessary to bake a cake in the toy kitchen, the clinician notes her excessive and abnormal dysfluencies. Alice not only has excessive repetitions, prolongations, and hesitations, but many of them are also abnormal—fundamentally different from the nonfluencies produced by normal speakers. But it is the struggle in Alice's speech that alarms the clinician. The child loses eye contact, contorts her face when trying to force an utterance, and even has tongue, lip, and jaw tremors, the most advanced sign of stuttering. Alice's pitch rises during utterances because of the increase in laryngeal muscular tension. Her speech is punctuated by gasping, with the ever-present schwa vowel *uh* between and within words. Never has the clinician seen such an advanced case of stuttering in such a young child.

After the evaluation is concluded, the two clinicians meet with Michelle in the conference room. Alice and the receptionist play in the Kid's Room while the results of the stuttering evaluation and treatment options are discussed with the anxious parent. The clinicians comment on Alice's remarkable language development and its possible role in her stuttering. They explain that some children stutter because their language development far exceeds their motor speech abilities. The result is a gap between language demands and speech production capabilities, and consequently, these children are excessively dysfluent. The clinicians also explain the role of an improper diagnosis of stuttering by parents and could make Alice self-conscious and anxious about her speech. This is done carefully, without casting blame. The clinicians conclude the diagnostic report with the observation that many factors may be involved in Alice's stuttering, including an inherited gene, and that possibly nothing could have prevented it. They also convey their optimism about the potential for successful treatment, especially since the problem was diagnosed early.

Over the next 2 years, Alice responds well to the prevention and treatment program. Initially, she is seen three times per week at the clinic and her parents are counseled weekly. Alice meets with a clinician in the Kid's Room and plays with the multitude of dolls, cars, kitchen devices, and games. The clinician works on improving Alice's speech-related self-esteem, removing speech anxiety, and increasing her tolerance and acceptance of dysfluent speech. Gradually, Alice's anxiety about speech fluency dwindles. During the first year, she continues to be excessively dysfluent, but as she matures neurologically, her speech becomes more and more fluent and eventually her language demands parallel her neuromotor speech capacity. At home, Alice's parents help remove unrealistic fluency expectations and create an environment where nonfluencies are expected, accepted, and, in some situations, even encouraged. When Alice starts school, the speech-language pathologist is notified of her stuttering history so that booster therapies can be provided if necessary. Fortunately, therapy is not necessary, and today Alice is a normally speaking 12-year-old with only vague memories of stuttering and the games she played in the Kid's Room at the speech and hearing clinic.

Case Study 3.2 An Individual with Mental Impairment–Mental Retardation Who Stutters

WALTER

Seventeen-year-old Walter does menial labor, and his primary job is to keep the Vintage Clothing Store stocked. Although Walter has a tested IQ of 63, he knows that the store is a big source of income for the Center for Human Development, which provides jobs, food, housing, and therapy for 12 mentally impaired–mentally retarded individuals.

Walter cannot remember when he first started stuttering; it seems he has stuttered all his life. He continues to have stuttering therapy three times per week provided by student therapists from the university, but over the years there has been little improvement in his speech. His case manager has made an appointment with a stuttering specialist to see if continued therapy is warranted. The specialist will decide if Walter can benefit from stuttering therapy, and if so, what programs will result in improvement.

Walter enters your office and takes a seat at the diagnostic table. You and the clean-cut teenager share a few pleasantries. The case manager's report states that Walter was first diagnosed with stuttering when he was 5 and has been seen by nearly 20 therapists since then. Initially, stuttering therapy was provided concurrently with language stimulation and literacy training. At about the time he entered middle school, it was decided that his language acquisition had plateaued and he had achieved his maximum literacy skills. Special education resources focused on eliminating his severe stuttering. The most recent fluency test showed him to have extremely severe stuttering with many accessory features.

During the many years of stuttering therapy, Walter has had every conceivable treatment. Early in the development of his stuttering, prevention strategies were used in the belief that he simply had many normal nonfluencies that he would eventually outgrow. Later, his speech was desensitized and modified, and he was taught to stutter fluently. He was encouraged to talk more slowly, breathe deeply, and pace his speech to a metronome. For a while, he even used a special hearing aid that helped only initially. When you read the report, you see that a well-intentioned physician suggested that clipping his lingual frenulum might be helpful. Fortunately, this surgery was not performed. Walter was prescribed muscle relaxants, but they did not help him talk more fluently; they simply caused him to be lethargic and were stopped. Finally, in a special conference with his parents, teachers, case managers, and social workers, it was agreed that a decision was needed on whether Walter would ever talk normally.

You have been authorized to make that determination, by which everyone involved in Walter's stuttering will abide. You have a week to make this important decision.

You conduct a series of evaluations. Walter is pleasant and cooperative as you try different therapies. You discover that he is unable to achieve any type of fluent speech for more than a few seconds. Try as he may, he simply cannot modify his speech consistently to reduce or eliminate the dysfluencies. You reward easy contacts, slower rates of speech, and even speaking with a southern drawl. You show Walter how to relax his speech muscles and how to make each sound easily and gently. But it is to no avail; Walter is incapable of a minimum of fluent speech even in a controlled clinical setting. No therapy can create the necessary level of fluency to be rewarded, expanded, and, hopefully, generalized.

Finally, in a last-ditch attempt, you set up a delayed auditory feedback (DAF) device. This instrument has settings allowing the speaker's auditory feedback to be delayed by a fraction of a second. You place the earphones over Walter's ears, set the delay to maximum, and have him discuss story pictures. Delayed auditory feedback causes normal speakers to be dysfluent; they have more repetitions, hesitations, and prolongations, and the longer the delay, the more dysfluent they are. Walter also displays increased dysfluencies because of the maximum delay. (You are disappointed that he does not have near-fluent speech, as do some persons who stutter under the conditions of DAF.) After allowing him to discuss the story pictures with the maximum auditory feedback delay, you gradually reduce the delay, hoping that Walter will have adjusted and consequently will be more fluent. Then, gradually, you can reduce the delay to real time. If the theory works with Walter, you will have the necessary fluent speech behaviors to reward. You have found that persons with low intelligence quotients respond better to behavior modification than to many other types of stuttering therapy, which require high levels of psychological and intellectual participation that are beyond the reach of many individuals with mental impairment–mental retardation. Using behavior modification, you can gradually get Walter to be more and more fluent in controlled situations, and hopefully, over time, generalize the behavior to all speaking situations.

Unfortunately, Walter is unable to achieve the level of fluency necessary for operant conditioning. Although he becomes more fluent by gradually reducing the DAF, it is not enough, nor can he maintain it, even when rewards are given for each fluent utterance. You try several variations of delaying the auditory feedback, but they too are unsuccessful. It appears that you, like the many previous clinicians, cannot make meaningful and persistent gains in Walter's speech fluency. You and Walter discuss your belief that stuttering therapy should be terminated permanently, and you find that he agrees. In your report, you state that the time has come for Walter to learn to accept his stuttering rather than trying futilely to overcome it.

Clinical Sidebar 3.2

Some persons think that society's attitude toward stuttering should be changed. They believe that many persons who stutter cannot significantly improve their fluency and that society should accept their speech. They point out that stuttering usually does not impair intelligibility, and that it should be viewed as simply a different speech pattern and not stigmatized. What do you think?

Case Study 3.3 Stuttering Therapy in a Camp Situation

The University Stuttering Camp has an excellent reputation. Affiliated with one of the largest universities in the Midwest, it is held in early August and provides 12 teenagers with 8 days of intensive stuttering therapy. Twelve student clinicians from the United States and Canada are selected from among many applicants to provide clinical services. There are two full-time clinical supervisors, and the program is directed by a visiting professor. Several volunteers, members of a national stuttering association, also attend. They take vacation time and leave from their jobs to help the campers with their stuttering problems. In addition, a large corporation has donated several computers and stuttering treatment programs. The campers, their parents, clinicians, and volunteers fly to the Midwest, taxi to the camp, and meet for the first time. A local television crew is on hand to capture the event.

The camp is located on 40 picturesque acres owned by a national service organization and provided to the university free of charge. It is on the outskirts of the city, nestled in the surrounding rolling hills with small farms. At the center of the camp is a large pavilion, a fire pit for the nightly campfires, a mess hall, and four rows of very small cottages. In the cottages, the campers, clinicians, and volunteers bunk. A small fish-filled creek runs through the property, and just down the dirt road is an ancient, huge red barn with a loft, horse stalls, and stacks of hay. Every day after the stuttering therapy sessions end, the director of the camp, supervisors, and clinicians meet at the barn and have lively discussions about stuttering theories and practices. Sitting on hay bales, the eager student clinicians discuss the joys and frustrations of stuttering therapy.

Each morning at 7:00 a.m., the camp is awakened by the ringing of the meal bell. The cottages gradually empty and sleepy people walk to the mess hall, where breakfast is served. At 8:15, the clinical staff meets in the pavilion to review the daily treatment objectives and the methods that will be used to achieve them. Because there are 12 graduate clinicians from 12 different universities, the therapies provided to the campers are an eclectic mix, tailored to each camper's unique history. Attempts are made to be consistent with the therapies provided to the campers before they came to the camp, but variation and experimentation are also encouraged.

At 9:00, campers and clinicians pair off for 3 hours of individual therapy. The sessions are conducted in the pavilion, the barn, and the cottages. Also, clinicians and campers simply walk the rolling hills, capture butterflies, and pick flowers; some even fish the creek. The director and supervisors supervise the sessions, but they are careful to remain in the background as much as possible. At noon, lunch is served in the mess hall. The director, supervisors, and clinicians eat in the pavilion, review and adjust the treatment plans, and discuss progress. The campers and volunteers eat together in the amphitheater a few yards from the cabins. After lunch, another hour of individual stuttering therapy is provided. Afterward, the campers and volunteers do what they have been eagerly anticipating: they take long hikes, shoot model rockets into the humid sky, practice hitting large targets with bows and arrows, play softball on a makeshift diamond, and do other enjoyable activities. The clinical staff meet in the barn and write treatment plans. After supper, movies are shown for the campers and volunteers in the amphitheater. They then play games and have lively discussions late into the evening. During the exit interviews, many campers remark that the time spent with the volunteers from the national stuttering association provided them with valuable insights and coping strategies. They also appreciated the fact that only the volunteers and campers spent that time together. One camper proudly remarked, "You had to be a stutterer" to be a member of that select group.

Clinical Sidebar 3.3

Many persons who stutter can become normally fluent in a controlled clinical environment. However, regardless of the therapeutic approach, carryover of what is learned in the clinic to real-life situations is an important part of successful treatment. To be successful, stuttering therapies must address the client's speech fluency outside of the clinic, including how fluently the person talks at home, in the classroom, on the playground, and so forth. Why is it unlikely that there will ever be a quick cure for stuttering?

Day 7 of the stuttering camp is eagerly anticipated by campers, volunteers, and clinical staff alike. At 10:00 a.m., several large vans enter the camp to take everyone to a large shopping mall. Located in the city, the mall is three stories tall, with hundreds of stores, eating establishments, video game rooms, skate boarding facilities, and even an ice rink. Clinicians and their clients pair off and go "trophy hunting"—an opportunity for the clients to use their fluency tools in real situations. The clients ask directions, request change, order food, and do all the things teenagers do at malls. However, they do them using easy contacts (light pressure), relaxed speech musculature, pullout devices (ways of not stuttering), and cancellations (stopping and starting over again using fluency tools). They concentrate on their respiration and prolong certain sounds, avoiding facial grimacing, hand slaps, head jerks, or tongue, jaw, and lip tremors. They have positive speaking attitudes and tolerance for their dysfluencies. They maintain eye contact. Most of the clients do these things remarkably well, and the clinical staff know that at least some generalization to real-life speaking situations has occurred.

"Captain Karen," as the campers call her, has been given leave from the Army to volunteer at the stuttering camp, and she and the campers have planned a "water gun war" all week. The scheme is for the campers to attack the volunteers and clinical staff after supper in a carefully designed raid. Captain Karen has brought Army camouflage uniforms, face paint, and tarps, and each camper has been issued a heavy-duty water gun capable of drenching the enemy in seconds. The campers can hardly be seen in the dusky light as they creep silently on their mission. They crawl on hands and knees, blending into the environment, sliding through the trees and bushes. Loud decoy music radiates from the amphitheater. Unsuspecting clinicians laugh outside their cottages, several volunteers encircle the beer cooler, and the director reviews the final reports for tomorrow's meeting with the campers' parents. The unsuspecting victims are enjoying the final night of the stuttering camp when the surprise attack occurs. The battle is quick and decisive, leaving the campers clearly victorious and more than a little pleased with themselves.

The next day, family members arrive and meet with the clinicians and volunteers. The director reviews each camper's progress and provides a written summary to be given to the client's therapist. The television news crew again interviews parents, clinicians, and campers, and by late afternoon, the picturesque 40 acres have returned to their original condition. Campers, volunteers, and clinical staff travel home with fond memories of 8 days well spent.

Case Study 3.4 A 22-Year-Old Man with Severe Anxiety-Based Stuttering

JUAN SEDILLO

Several therapy sessions were devoted to listing the most stressful and anxiety-provoking sounds, words, situations, and persons in Juan Sedillo's life. Juan carefully identified and placed them in descending order. At the top of the "sound" list was the horrid *b* sound, which caused his lips to purse tightly and tremor. But it was the closing of his vocal cords that completely prohibited him from making that dreaded sound. With his lips and vocal cords tightly closed, Juan had to wait for the *b* sound to slide reluctantly from his mouth. And it seemed that the more he forced the sound, the more it resisted. Over the years, Juan had come to hate this sound.

Juan's most feared and anxiety-provoking "word" was his name. Time after time when asked, "Name please?" Juan felt the word stick in his throat. Nothing could be more embarrassing, and it seemed that everyone demanded his name. From the clerk at Radio Shack to his barber, "Name please?" was a frequent request. For Juan, the most distressing aspect of stuttering was being unable to say his own name. Even a toddler could do that! Just thinking about the surprised expressions on people's faces and their mean comments caused Juan to cringe. There always seemed to be a budding comedian showing off to everyone in earshot: "Cat got your tongue?"

At the top of the feared and anxiety-provoking "situation" list was the telephone. For Juan, there was no question that answering the telephone prompted stuttering. It happened every time the telephone rang, and shivers shot down his spine as he answered it. He knew that when he picked it up, he had to speak immediately. If he did not, he would hear "Hello, hello . . . is someone there?" Of course, this caused him even more trouble in speaking, and often the caller would hang up in mid-stutter. A few seconds later, the phone would ring again, with a rerun of the sad comedy.

Juan liked his boss, and he was sure that the feeling was mutual. However, she was at the top of his distressing "people" list. After graduating from college with a degree in robotic engineering, Juan had landed a job at a local engineering company. Although the interview was a disaster (job interviews ranked second on his situation list), he was hired on the spot. In today's job market, engineering graduates, especially those in robotics, can choose their jobs, even if they have a stutter. His boss was in her 40s and reminded him of his mother. Although she had never talked about his speech disorder, Juan knew she empathized with him. Lately, she had begun helping him talk during stuttering moments, but that

Clinical Sidebar 3.4

Temporal urgency is the need to do something in a hurry. With few exceptions, speech temporal urgency causes persons who stutter to do so frequently and severely. Provide several ways of relieving temporal urgency in a person who stutters.

only seemed to make matters worse. Certainly, there were times when it was helpful for a friendly cue to say a word, but most of the time, all he really wanted was uninterrupted time to speak.

Juan also liked his new clinician. He seemed to know several theories about stuttering and was very good about explaining them. Sometimes, however, Juan felt that he knew more about this communication disorder than even the most knowledgeable specialist. After all, he had been in therapy most of his life.

The new clinician was working on desensitizing Juan to the stimuli that prompt stuttering. He explained that if the anxiety and negative emotions associated with sounds, words, situations, and certain people are removed, the stuttering can also be reduced or eliminated. That was the theory behind this treatment approach. Unfortunately, Juan knew that in stuttering therapy, what seemed to be workable in theory often did not succeed in practice. But Juan was an optimist, and he was doing his best.

It was true that certain sounds, words, situations, and persons triggered anxiety and muscle tightness in Juan. For many years, he had felt out of control when trying to talk and had suffered the ever-present embarrassment of stuttering. He had come to expect the anxiety and associated negative emotions when stuttering occurred. When speaking, he would scan ahead, searching for approaching stuttering cues. Sometimes he could avoid them, but most of the time there was no alternative but to forge ahead and suffer the anxiety and embarrassment.

The clinician explained that there were several ways of desensitizing Juan to stuttering stimuli. The idea was to pair neutral or positive emotions with the previously learned negative ones. Because of these pairings, gradually the negative emotions would be minimized or eliminated. The process of desensitization would begin with the least anxious and negative stimuli on Juan's lists and gradually move to the top. According to the clinician, there were several ways of creating the requisite neutral or positive emotions to be used for conditioning.

One way of creating these emotions was by medication. Juan had been prescribed Valium for his stutter when he was younger, and he did not like that option. He knew that antianxiety medications are habit-forming, and he disliked the negative effects such as drowsiness and lethargy. He also did not like to use a biofeedback device to achieve neutral or positive emotions for counterconditioning. Learning to relax muscles to the beeping of a tone seemed artificial. Of all the options, Juan most preferred progressive relaxation, autohypnosis, and meditation on a taped program. The clinician had provided him with individual instruction on the process and a tape that he could use at home.

In desensitization therapy, Juan came to the clinic 1 hour early. In the "relaxation room," he sat in an overstuffed chair and listened to the announcer's voice on the relaxation tape. The announcer instructed him to alternately tense and relax various body parts. Starting with his feet and systematically working up to his speech muscles, the announcer had Juan concentrate on groups of muscles and how to relax them. He also had Juan focus on his relaxation word to the exclusion of other verbal thoughts and told him to imagine serene, tranquil scenes. During the exercise, Juan took deep breaths and gradually exhaled while sensing the tension leave his body. At the conclusion of the 50-minute tape, the announcer counted backward from 10 and, with each number, suggested that Juan felt even higher levels of relaxation and a sensation of well-being. Juan also used the tape each evening and sometimes during his lunch hour. In therapy, he was being taught how to group muscles and to achieve the same levels of relaxation in an abbreviated way. The clinician wanted him to be able to relax his body, and particularly his speech muscles, in 2 to 3 minutes. Most importantly, the clinician wanted Juan to not allow his anxiety and tension to increase to high levels while stuttering.

In previous sessions, Juan had been deconditioned to the ringing of the telephone. Initially, he sat and simply listened to it ring. Later, he practiced relaxing his body, particularly his speech muscles, while walking to answer it. Today, Juan is being desensitized while talking on the telephone. The clinician has removed a telephone from its jack, and Juan is talking while holding the dead receiver to his ear. In the past, Juan reflexively tightened his muscles and felt a deep sense of dread and anxiety about talking on the telephone, but today he is doing it with positive emotions and relaxed speech muscles. As an added deconditioning goal, Juan is using the top five anxious and feared words on his list in sentences. In future sessions, Juan will make telephone calls to friends, relatives, and business acquaintances while maintaining positive psychological and physical states.

During the 6-month course of stuttering therapy, Juan became desensitized to the sounds, words, situations, and persons on his lists. Each of these stimuli gradually lost its ability to create anxiety and associated negative emotions. Loss of their power to cause stuttering, combined with talking with relaxed speech muscles and using other fluency-enhancing methods, allowed Juan to control his communication disorder. Juan did not like using the word *cure* to describe the results of therapy because when he was tired or distracted, he sometimes slipped back into the old patterns of stimulus-response stuttering. However, most of the time, he could control his stutter. His victory over anxiety and verbal impotence was apparent when Juan called his boss, requested an appointment, and successfully negotiated a hefty raise—all without significant stuttering.

Case Study 3.5 Preventing Stuttering in a 5-Year-Old Boy

STEVEN

Steven started stuttering when he was just 5 years old. It was the kindergarten "show and tell" fiasco that had devastated him. Afterward, his mother came to school and took him home. He spent the rest of that memorable day in his room playing with toys and watching television. As usual, the next morning, he rode the bus to school, but things had changed. A schoolmate was now calling him "Stuttering Steven." He dreaded returning to the classroom.

Fall was in the air, and Steven enjoyed capturing the bug for show and tell. He found a yellow caterpillar hiding in the red and orange leaves under the big oak tree in his backyard. It had more legs than he could count, and he carefully placed it in a jar with breathing holes punched in the top, pulling grass and clover and carefully putting them in the jar along with his crawly prize. He could hardly wait until tomorrow's show and tell.

Clinical Sidebar 3.5

Parents sometimes believe that it is helpful to remind their children not to stutter. While this is well intentioned, causing the child to be self-conscious about speech can exacerbate the fluency problem. Parents should be attentive, patient, and try to ignore their child's dysfluencies. If the child expresses concern about his or her speech fluency, the parent should say that all children occasionally have trouble with their speech and that the problem is likely temporary. What are some speech behaviors in a child suggesting that the parents should seek a stuttering evaluation?

All summer long, Steven's mother had been concerned about his speech. She first noted his stutter when the ice cream truck travelled through the neighborhood. Steven and his friends came running to their mothers, begging for money. Steven stuttered while asking for it, and even his friends looked at him with quizzical expressions. Several times, Steven's mother told him to slow down and think before speaking, and she reminded him not to stutter. She tried to hide her impatience and her growing concern about her son's speech disorder, but found it more and more difficult as the summer progressed.

On the morning of show and tell, Steven placed the jar with the bug in his backpack. The bus ride to school was uneventful, and soon he had taken his seat in Mrs. Lawson's kindergarten classroom. Student after student brought their objects to the front of the class and proudly discussed them. At the end of each presentation, Mrs. Lawson lavished praise on them for a job well done. Finally it was Steven's turn. He carefully shook the jar so that everyone could see the colorful bug. The class responded with awe as he pulled it from the jar and allowed everyone to take a closer look. Then he replaced it and began the telling part of show and tell.

Mrs. Lawson was concerned about Steven participating in show and tell. She suspected he was starting to stutter, but knew little about the disorder and how to prevent it. Several times in the past, he had stuttered while asking for directions and appeared unable to control his speech. The other children in the class seemed to be aware of his difficulties, and several boys were starting to make fun of him. Mrs. Lawson did not know what to do about show and tell. Should she exclude him or would that draw even more attention to his stuttering? She decided to allow him to participate and hoped for the best. Unfortunately, show and tell turned out to be a disaster for Steven.

Mrs. Lawson asked Steven to describe the circumstances surrounding the bug's capture. Steven said, "I found, I found, I . . . , uh . . . , I found, I found, I . . ." There was uncomfortable rustling in the classroom, and he tried again. "I found. I . . ., uh . . ." He tried repeatedly to speak, but to no avail. Mrs. Lawson did not know what to do or say. Again Steven tried to talk about oak trees, colorful oak leaves, and autumn evenings, but his lips seemed paralyzed. Another boy in the classroom said something about "Porky Pig," and the class burst into laughter. Mrs. Lawson watched as Steven stopped talking and began to cry. She helped him to his seat and announced that the class should prepare for lunch. She told Steven that he had a fine bug in the jar and it was a great addition to show and tell. Steven asked to see the school nurse, and Mrs. Lawson walked with the crying youngster to the nurse's station.

Two weeks later, the speech-language pathologist, Mrs. Lawson, and other educational professionals met with Steven's mother to discuss what could be done about his stutter. The therapist had previously attended several classes and observed Steven interact with the teacher and other pupils. The clinician also provided Mrs. Lawson and Steven's mother with a questionnaire on his speech fluency in the classroom and at home. Everyone at the meeting agreed that his dysfluencies exceeded the norm, and that Steven was self-conscious and anxious about speaking. However, they believed that it was not too late to prevent him from becoming a lifelong stutterer.

Mrs. Lawson and the speech therapist met regularly to discuss ways to remove stress while speaking and to minimize Steven's self-consciousness about his dysfluencies. During this critical period of prevention, Mrs. Lawson designed classroom activities that did not require Steven to speak publicly or to answer questions, and she did this without drawing negative attention to him. She also met with the pupil who was making fun of Steven's speech and encouraged him to stop. Steven's mother was counseled to remove speaking stress at home and not to draw attention to his speech dysfluencies.

In accordance with the IEP, the speech clinician did not remove Steven from the classroom to work on his speech fluency. Pullout therapy, it was believed, would draw attention to his problem and make him more self-conscious. The therapist regularly came to the classroom and worked with Steven on classroom assignments and on his speech. Steven was praised for speech fluency and encouraged to talk easily and without force. His speech-related self-esteem was bolstered by frequent statements such as "Excellent talking," "I like how you said that," "You certainly have good things to say," and "Great speaking." With the help of Steven's mother, Mrs. Lawson, and the speech clinician, Steven lost his self-consciousness about his speech fluency and stopped struggling to talk. Eventually, the memories of that disturbing show and tell faded. He was monitored throughout elementary school for relapse and eventually began middle school as a normal-speaking youngster.

Case Study 3.6   The Role of Stuttering Therapy Secondary Gains in a Male College Student

CHAD

Linda suspected that Chad, her first client with a stutter, was attracted to her, and she did not know how to handle it. Linda is a second-year graduate student in speech-language pathology with most of her courses completed. This semester, she is seeing clients at the university's speech and hearing clinic and looking forward to her off-campus externship next term. Most of her supervised clinical activities are in the afternoon, and three times a week at 3:00 p.m., she greets Chad in the waiting room. Together they walk to the stuttering therapy suite and work on his mild stutter. Chad has been a client of the clinic for several years, and Linda, like many clinicians before her, is not making a significant, long-lasting improvement. Chad can achieve normal fluency in the clinic, but there is no carryover to outside situations. What is even more frustrating is that Chad appears to be more and more disturbed by his fluency disorder.

During a conference, Linda's clinical supervisor states that Chad may be gaining secondarily from stuttering therapy, which is contributing to the poor clinical results. The supervisor suggests that perhaps Chad craves the interaction with female student clinicians and that stuttering therapy is becoming a social activity. The supervisor thinks that, either consciously or subconsciously, Chad resists speech improvement because he knows that the sessions will end and he will no longer be able to enjoy the interaction with the clinicians. It is also possible that the clinicians' professional concern and empathy for Chad also provide secondary gains. Apparently, Chad has few social outlets and no family support.

Chad began going to the university's speech and hearing clinic as a freshman and has been in therapy ever since. He is soon to graduate, and even the thought of job interviews makes him nervous. He looks forward to the sessions and wishes they could be held daily. The only criticism Chad has about the services at the clinic is the lack of consistency. Every clinician starts from scratch, going over the same things addressed by previous clinicians and making no improvement until the latter part of the semester. This semester his student clinician is Linda, and she is the best therapist yet. He plans to ask the supervisor if she can be his clinician next semester.

Chad has always been awkward with people. As a teenager, he suffered from the usual adolescent angst, particularly around girls. It was difficult to muster the courage to sit near them during lunch period or to participate in study groups. And like most boys, he needed great courage and resolve to ask a girl out for a date and to deal with real or imagined rejection. Chad struggled during high school in dealing with girls, and his stutter was a serious complication. For example, during school dances, Chad found the courage to take the "long walk" to the opposite side of the dance floor, politely ask a classmate to dance, and, like most boys, anticipate the possibility of rejection. But unlike many boys, Chad, because of his stutter, wore his anxiety on his sleeve. Frequently, he suffered the inevitable smiles, jokes, and mean comments of those nearby. Chad weathered the rejection of high school and eventually entered college.

Because of Chad's stuttering, college was not much different from high school. He still had problems dealing with the opposite sex. It wasn't that college women were rude; he simply couldn't find the courage to walk up to them and start a conversation. He tried many ways, including having his roommate approach them first and explain that Chad would be asking for a date. He tried blind dates and a computer dating service offered by student government. Meeting women in bars and at parties was a disaster. He even tried first confessing that he stuttered and then attempting to start a conversation. But apparently, nothing could overcome the stuttering obstacle to meeting women. After 3 years of college, Chad preferred to be lonely than to suffer rejection. At least for 3 hours a week, he could talk to Linda about his life, fears, anxiety, and stuttering. He cherished the weekly sessions and talking to a thoughtful, caring person. Sometimes he wondered what he would do without stuttering therapy.

Linda and her clinical supervisor discussed ways to make Chad less dependent on stuttering therapy and to remove the potential for secondary gains. First, they agreed to encourage Chad to go to the counseling center. A counselor, with an understanding of stuttering, could help Chad deal with his social interaction problems and ego restriction. The clinical supervisor explained to Linda that ego restriction, a concept developed by Anna Freud, occurs when a person unnecessarily limits his or her life rather than suffer potential rejection. Ego restriction is an aspect of an inferiority complex. Second, they agreed that Linda would continue to act professionally toward Chad and not allow the relationship to develop beyond the therapy sessions. On several occasions, Chad had asked her to have coffee with him after the session, and once he asked her to a movie. Third, they agreed that Chad had to take a greater role in planning and directing his therapy. He needed to identify his objectives, how to achieve them, and what criteria would be used to decide when they had been met. Finally, a date for termination of therapy would be set if progress could not be demonstrated. Although Chad would resist, Linda and her supervisor agreed that it was the only ethical course to take.

Linda and her supervisor met with Chad and discussed the long-term objectives of his therapy. At first, Chad disagreed with their assessment and the need to discontinue therapy if no progress could be demonstrated. He also questioned whether he was gaining secondarily from the sessions. Eventually, he agreed to the changes in the long-term objectives and actively participated in the design and procedures of his stuttering program. He met regularly with a counselor from the counseling and testing center. The following semester, Chad suggested that his stuttering therapy gradually be reduced and stopped by the end of the term. His stutter had diminished significantly outside the clinical setting, and what remained of it was tolerable to him. Thanks to counseling, his self-esteem had improved dramatically, and combined with the reduction in stuttering, Chad no longer felt socially hindered. He graduated from college and moved to a large city where his occasional mild stutter did not unduly restrict his social life.

Case Study 3.7   Integrating Transactional Analysis Counseling into Stuttering Therapy

CLARENE

Clarene works for the medical division of a large corporation. The company is a national leader in heart valve and artery transplants. With a degree in microbiology,

Clarene's first and only job has been with this prestigious corporation. One of her responsibilities is to run tests using the scanning electron microscope. Animal tissue is sent to her lab, and she uses a state-of-the-art microscope and other instruments to look for tissue degradation and signs of rejection. Her job is exciting and demanding, and she looks forward to the daily challenges.

Clinical Sidebar 3.7
In stuttering therapy, there are two general approaches to counseling the client: directive and controlled nondirective. In directive counseling, the clinician acts as the leader in helping the client work through the psychological issues associated with stuttering. In controlled nondirective counseling, such as is practiced in Transactional Analysis, the client decides when and how to address the psychological issues while the clinician probes, reflects, and provides feedback. Which type of counseling do you believe will produce the best results for persons who stutter?

It has been nearly 10 years since Clarene completed stuttering therapy. As she recalls the years of therapy she endured, she realizes that stuttering, like many of life's adversities, has made her a better person. Certainly, the stuttering-related rejection and embarrassment she suffered while growing up added layers of maturational difficulty, but because of them, she learned a lot about herself and others. In her early 20s, she was introduced to a counseling approach known as Transactional Analysis, (TA) which still provides a philosophy that teaches her how to deal with stuttering and other important life issues. This counseling approach was developed by Eric Berne and gained widespread popularity in the latter 20th century. Even today, Clarene uses the Transactional Analysis concepts she learned in stuttering therapy in addressing relationship issues and occasional feelings of inferiority, especially those related to speech. Transactional Analysis uses words easily understood and descriptive of psychological concepts; it is not fettered by unnecessary psychiatric jargon. It is based on research showing that most experiences stored in a person's mind can be retrieved, along with the feelings associated with them. On a day-to-day basis, those memories, good and bad, are called up, forming and influencing the thoughts, attitudes, feelings, and behaviors of adults. According to Transactional Analysis, there are three components of the personality: Child, Parent, and Adult.

Clarene is happy to know that the Child in her personality is alive and well. This part of her ego has both natural and adapted components. The part of her personality that needs and seeks affection, acceptance, total freedom, and love is the Natural Child. This aspect of the Child holds Clarene's memories of her first grand experiences with life and her feelings associated with them. It is curious and desires to explore the world.

The Adapted Child is the negative component of Clarene's personality, and unfortunately, she knows that it too is alive and well. The Adapted Child represents frustration and other negative experiences associated with the socialization process. It is the Adapted Child who conformed to the wishes of her parents and teachers; it is passive, inadequate, inferior, and clumsy. For Clarene, the Adapted Child represents memories of having speech that was "too little this or too much that." Stuttering was born in the Adapted Child. Sometimes, simply a word, touch, odor, or image can stimulate stored images, internal monologues, and the feelings associated with the Adapted Child psychological state, and they are the source of Clarene's feelings about some speaking situations. In Transactional Analysis terminology, her Adapted Child is *snagged* by certain cues.

The Parent component of Clarene's personality consists of regulating and nurturing forces. It consists of thoughts, feelings, and attitudes learned from her parents and parent substitutes such as the church and school, the "shoulds" and "should-nots" taught to children by authority figures. As Clarene has learned, the Parent part of her personality leads her to think and act as her parents (or parent substitutes) would want her to do. There are two aspects to Clarene's Parent: the Critical Parent and Nurturing Parent ego states.

Clarene's Critical Parent consists of the controlling, directing aspects of her personality. This ego state continues to regulate some of her thoughts, attitudes, and behaviors and causes a feeling of inadequacy. While growing up, Clarene was subjected to many critical directives and comments about speech fluency, and those thoughts and feelings are still with her.

The Nurturing Parent ego state reduces anxiety and makes the Child feel comfortable and loved. This part of Clarene's personality provides comfort in much the same way as her actual parents. Unfortunately, for Clarene, there are few nurturing statements from childhood about her communication disorder.

The Adult part of Clarene's personality is like a computer; it is unemotional and operates on facts, statistics, and objective information. This ego state is in contact with reality and can reevaluate old messages imprinted on Clarene when she was a child. It tests the reality of her current thinking patterns and accepts or rejects the earlier-learned information. In well-adjusted persons, the Adult is fully developed by the early teens and begins the lifelong process of assessing reality. However, for Clarene, it took longer for her Adult to develop and examine the outdated early information about speaking and stuttering, and to assess it from the viewpoint of a mature woman. With the benefit of counseling, she learned to reject the Adapted Child's thoughts and feelings about her speech. Transactional Analysis taught her how to understand and reduce the feeling of inferiority from which she suffered for so many years.

Clarene learned that without the benefit of an active Adult, outdated and unrealistic thoughts can permeate a person's life. The person who stutters can feel overwhelmed by negative thoughts about speaking and other social activities that were learned as a child, and these patterned ways of thinking can become strong habits. The Adult in Clarene's personality allows her to reject those thoughts and feelings about speaking and to adopt the belief that her speech is acceptable and natural. She no longer allows herself to feel like that young girl who was subjected to so many negative attitudes in connection with speaking. Clarene simply makes the conscious (Adult) decision that she and her speech are acceptable and natural, and does not allow herself to be saturated with embarrassment, shame, guilt, and anxiety about speaking.

Another benefit of Transactional Analysis was learning that other persons also have Parent, Adult, and Child aspects of their personalities. When communication transactions are complementary—that is, when both parties communicate from the same ego states, such as Child-Child, Adult-Adult, or Parent-Parent, or, for example, when the Adapted Child in one party seeks the Nurturing Parent in the other—then the communication is satisfying and rewarding. However, when uncomplementary or crossed transactions occur, communication breaks down and both parties feel negative and misunderstood. Communication, the foundation of relationships, becomes unsatisfying and unproductive.

Clarene understands that Transactional Analysis does not work for all persons to address the social and psychological aspects of stuttering. There are many counseling approaches and ways of gaining insight into this potentially devastating communication disorder. However, for Clarene, Transactional Analysis provides a means of exploring her thoughts and feelings about stuttering. It also provides a way of understanding communication with others that has benefited her in developing and maintaining intimate and business relationships. Clarene sometimes believes that having a stutter has been a blessing in disguise.

SUMMARY

Stuttering is a fluency disorder in which an individual repeats, prolongs, and blocks while speaking. There also may be ancillary (secondary features) such eye squints, hand slaps, and head jerks. Many persons who stutter report anxiety and associated negative emotions before, during, and after the moment of stuttering. There are many theories about stuttering, but none of them is generally accepted as the sole cause of this communication disorder. In most cases, stuttering is more easily prevented than cured. To reduce or eliminate stuttering, its audible and visible manifestations, as well as the anxiety and associated negative emotions, must be treated, in addition to addressing the effects of the disorder on the client's self-concept and speech-related self-esteem.

Study and Discussion Questions

1. Discuss Van Riper's definition of stuttering. How might you expand it to include more aspects of stuttering?

2. Discuss the important issues in the nature-nurture controversy about stuttering.

3. List and describe the organic theories of stuttering.

4. List and describe the psychological theories of stuttering.

5. List and describe the learning theories of stuttering.

6. How might stuttering be caused by multiple etiological factors?

7. Describe the diagnostic categories and treatment approaches for a child with a suspected fluency disorder.

8. Why might a false-positive diagnosis be more harmful than a false-negative one?

9. What are the audible symptoms of stuttering and some therapeutic approaches?

10. What are the visible features of stuttering and some therapeutic approaches?

11. How can speech-related anxiety and the associated negative emotions be desensitized?

12. Is there a stuttering personality? What role might stuttering play in the development of personality?

Recommended Reading

Tanner, D. (1994). *Pragmatic stuttering intervention for children* (2nd ed.) Oceanside, CA: Academic Communication Associates.

Tanner, D., Belliveau, W., & Siebert, G. (1995). *Pragmatic stuttering intervention for adolescents and adults.* Oceanside, CA: Academic Communication Associates.

These two stuttering programs address the four factors associated with stuttering and emphasize a variety of communication functions and acts.

Tanner, D. (1999). *Understand stuttering: A guide for parents.* Oceanside, CA: Academic Communication Associates.

This pamphlet describes stuttering and provides helpful suggestions for parents and teachers.

Tanner, D. (2003). *Exploring communication disorders: A 21st century introduction through literature and media.* Boston: Allyn & Bacon.

This book has a chapter on stuttering and uses references to literature and media to introduce and explain the communication disorder.

Yeoman, B. (1998, November–December). Wrestling with words. *Psychology Today, 31*(6), 42–47.

This article provides an alternative view of stuttering as a disorder. It suggests that some persons should learn to accept stuttering rather than striving to overcome it.

CHAPTER FOUR

Voice and Resonance Disorders

I'm exhausted from not talking.

Sam Goldwyn

Chapter Preview: In this chapter, voice and resonance impairments are discussed as a combined category of communication disorders. There is an overview of the speech resonating system and a discussion of the anatomy and physiology of voice production. The mechanics of phonation is examined, and voice qualities are critiqued. Voice and resonance disorders arising from cleft lip and palate, paralysis, laryngeal cancer and other diseases, vocal strain and abuse, and psychological factors are discussed. Because of the wide variety of voice disorders, factors related to diagnosis and treatment are addressed in each etiological category. Case studies are presented of total laryngectomy, unilateral adductor paralysis, vocal nodules, psychogenic aphonia, disorders related to laryngeal tissue scarring, and cleft lip and palate.

OVERVIEW OF VOICE AND RESONANCE DISORDERS

The human **larynx**, or voice box, is located in the neck and serves as an energy source for speech communication. The energy generated from the larynx, and to a lesser extent from other speech structures, **resonates** throughout the vocal tract, giving each speaker's voice its individual quality. The laryngeal sound source and the resonance potential of the head and neck cavities combine to produce the physical properties and psychological qualities of a person's speech and voice. Consequently, in this chapter, the discussion of voice disorders is not limited to laryngeal dysfunctions but also includes resonance disorders such as those that occur with cleft palate.

The Human Sound Source-Resonating System

One way of looking at the speech mechanism is to compare it to a musical instrument. In a trombone, for example, the player places the mouthpiece, the sound source, against the lips and makes a buzzing sound. The air and the trombone are set into vibration corresponding to the frequency and intensity of the sound. Certain frequencies of the buzzing sound are **amplified** or **damped** by the trombone, and the player changes the pitch by altering the frequency of the buzzing and by adjusting the length of the resonating chamber with the slide; the pitch decreases when the slide is extended. The trombone sounds like a trombone because of its shape, its texture, and the adjustable length of the resonating chamber. All musical instruments work in a similar sound source-resonating manner. They operate on the same principle whether the sound source is the buzzing of a reed, the vibration of a violin string, air turbulence over the mouth opening of a flute, or the hammering of a piano string. Some instruments have valves that open and close, changing the length of the resonating tube.

The voice production mechanism works in the same way as a musical instrument. The main sound source is the vibration of the vocal cords. Air pressure builds up below the vocal cords, and when it is great enough to overcome the **muscular resistance** and **static air** in the vocal tract, the cords are blown apart. They would stay apart if it were not for an **aerodynamic force** and **muscular elasticity**. The aerodynamic force is the **Bernoulli principle**, which accounts for a suction effect bringing the vocal cords together. **Elasticity** is the tendency of tissue to regain its original shape when stretched and distended. The suction effect of the Bernoulli principle and the tendency of the muscles and tissues in the larynx to regain their original shape after being stretched and distended allow the vocal folds to vibrate very rapidly. This **myoelastic-aerodynamic principle** of vocal fold vibration accounts for the ability of the vocal cords to vibrate extremely rapidly and not to fatigue over time.

The rate of vocal cord vibration is called the **fundamental frequency** and is the prime determinant of a person's **pitch**, the psychological perception of frequency of vibration. Although frequency and pitch are related, there is no one-to-one relationship between them; a unit increase or decrease in frequency does not necessarily correspond to the same subjective change in pitch.

Anatomy and Physiology of the Larynx

The larynx can be viewed as a **valve** that opens for breathing and closes when foods and liquids enter the throat. The larynx consists of nine **cartilages**, three of which are paired. (See Figure 4.1 for anterior and posterior views of the larynx.) The epiglottis, cricoid, and thyroid are the unpaired cartilages. The epiglottis closes over the larynx during swallowing to provide protection. It is helpful but not essential to a safe swallow. The cricoid cartilage resembles a signet ring and is located below the thyroid cartilage. The thyroid cartilage is the largest, and the "Adam's apple" is its anterior prominence.

The arytenoid, corniculate, and cuneiform are paired cartilages. The arytenoids are shaped like a pyramid and are important to pitch change. They slide, rock, and rotate and are primary structures in **abduction** (opening) or **adduction** (closing) of the vocal folds. The cuneiforms are wedge-shaped, and the corniculates are small cartilages attached to the apex (upper part) of the arytenoids. **Cranial nerve X**, also known as the **vagus** nerve, innervates, abducts, and adducts the vocal folds.

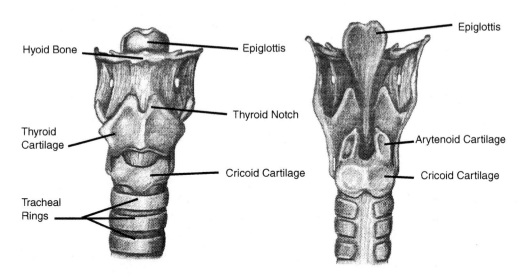

Figure 4.1 Anterior and posterior views of the larynx.

There are two types of laryngeal muscles: **extrinsic** and **intrinsic**. Extrinsic laryngeal muscles have their origin outside of the larynx and are sometimes called *neck strap muscles.* Extrinsic muscles may also be classified by their location, superior (suprahyoid) or inferior (infrahyoid) to the hyoid bone. The extrinsic laryngeal muscles are generally responsible for support of the larynx because it does not rest on a bone. They also move the larynx up or down during speech and swallowing. The intrinsic laryngeal muscles have both their origin and their attachment within the larynx. The **abductor** muscle, the posterior cricoarytenoid muscle, is primarily responsible for opening the **glottis**, the opening at the level of the larynx. The lateral cricoarytenoid, transverse arytenoid, and oblique arytenoid muscles are the primary **adductors** of the vocal folds (Stemple, 1984; Zemlin, 1998). During voicing, respiratory support is adjusted for the **impedance** (resistance) in the larynx; when the impedance to airflow changes, there is a consequent adjustment in respiratory support. Without respiratory support adjustments, utterances would have inappropriate pitch and loudness changes.

Age and Gender Differences in Phonation

The vocal cords vibrate very rapidly, and the vibratory sound produced at the level of the larynx is called **phonation**. In women, the vocal cords vibrate about 250 cycles per second, and in men, about 130 cycles per second. The vocal cords vibrate more frequently in women because the female larynx tends to be smaller and is usually shaped somewhat differently from that in men. This difference in laryngeal shape also contributes to the prominent thyroid notch in many men. In addition, Zemlin (1998) notes that with increasing age, the laryngeal cartilages tend to ossify, contributing to pitch alterations and airway resistance, which are greater in women than in men. According to Kent (1997), besides having

Table 4.1 Variables Affecting Pitch

Variable*	Effect on Fundamental Frequency (fo)
Increase mass/unit length	Lower pitch
Decrease mass/unit length	Increase pitch
Increase vocal fold tension	Increase pitch
Decrease vocal fold tension	Decrease pitch
Increase subglottal air pressure (P_{sub})	Increase pitch
Decrease subglottal air pressure (P_{sub})	Decrease pitch

*When all other variables are held constant.

a higher pitch, women tend to have a breathy voice quality. From about age 4 to 10 years, the fundamental frequency is stable and typically the same for both boys and girls. At about age 12, the male fundamental frequency changes and remains about one octave below that of the female (Kent, 1997). **Falsetto**, the extreme upper limit of the pitch range, occurs in both men and lower-pitched women (Zemlin, 1998). With advanced age, there is typically a small increase in male fundamental frequency, while in women, there is a small decrease.

Pitch-Changing Mechanism

The pitch-changing mechanism is a complex interaction between respiratory support and laryngeal activities (see Table 4.1). Several variables affect pitch. Adjustments affecting the **mass per unit length** of the vocal folds account for decreases and increases in fundamental frequency. When the mass per unit length of the vocal folds increases, the vocal folds become thicker and shorter, with a consequent decrease in pitch. Conversely, when the mass per unit length of the vocal folds decreases, the vocal folds become thinner and longer, with a consequent increase in pitch. **Vocal fold tension** also affects pitch; relative increases and decreases in tension result in corresponding increases and decreases in pitch. Finally, when all other variables are held constant, an increase in **subglottal air pressure** increases pitch and vice versa.

Velopharyngeal Functioning

Although all sounds produced by the speech mechanism have a degree of **nasal resonance**, in English three sounds are considered nasals: /m/, /n/, and ng (as in *thong*). They result from opening the **velopharyngeal port** and allowing air and the acoustic energy generated from the larynx to pass through the nasal chambers. With the port opened, the lips occlude the airstream in the production of the /m/ phoneme and the /n/ sound by the tip of the tongue approximating the alveolar ridge. The ng nasal is produced by opening the velopharyngeal port and the airstream occlusion by the back of the tongue approximating the **velum** (soft palate). The velum operates in binary mode, whereby the nerves and muscles function to either open or close the velopharyngeal port. In addition, in many speakers, the back of the pharynx contracts to create a bulge or pad to aid velopharyngeal closure. Some speakers have a distinct nasal quality to their speech and singing. This is normal and is simply a result of their unique velopharyngeal functioning and head and neck resonance characteristics.

Voice Quality

Speech is a stream of acoustic energy, and because it is intangible, descriptions of its **quality** vary greatly. The public uses a variety of terms to describe voice quality. A person's voice may be described as *tinny, throaty, sexy, metallic, hard, husky,* and so forth. Many of these terms are ill-defined and have little clinical use. Clinically, eight terms are used to describe the voice: **hypernasality**, **hyponasality**, **harsh**, **breathy**, **hoarse**, **hard glottal attack**, **strangled**, and **vocal fry**.

Hypernasality and hyponasality are voice qualities caused by abnormalities of the velopharyngeal port and nasal passageways. Hypernasality is too much nasality on non-nasal sounds. It occurs when the velopharyngeal port is open too long in connected speech or when there is a hole in the palates. It also occurs when the velum is too short or too small to approximate the posterior pharyngeal wall. Hyponasality, also called **denasality**, occurs when there is too little nasality on nasal sounds and the person appears to have an occluded nasal passageway.

A harsh voice quality occurs when the vocal cords close with too much force. Breathiness occurs for the opposite reason or when the period of closure is very brief. The hoarse voice is a result of uneven closure of the glottis; perceptually, it is a combination of harsh and breathy qualities. Some persons with a hoarse voice quality have mainly a breathy component, while others have more harshness.

Hard glottal attack resembles harshness; however, the forced closure occurs only on the initial sounds or syllables of words. The strangled voice quality is similar to harshness and sounds as though speech is being produced with extremely tense neck muscles. (Some patients have mucous buildup in the speech tract, giving the strained, strangled voice a "wet" quality.) The vocal fry voice quality is also known as *glottal fry*. The voice is low-pitched and pulsating, sometimes described as **creaking**.

Humans are marvelous sensing creatures, and the quality of a person's voice signals many personality traits and emotional states. According to Gobl and Ni' Chasaide (2002), there is no one-to-one mapping between voice quality and affect; instead, a given voice quality tends to be associated with a cluster of affective attributes. The nonverbal cues of a person's voice can carry as much communication information as the actual words—and sometimes more. In addition, if there is a conflict between the verbal and nonverbal information, the listener will usually believe the latter: "How something is spoken often speaks louder than what is said."

Cleft Lip and Palate

During the early weeks of pregnancy, the fetus's palatal shelves and nasal structures fuse. In about 1 in 700 live births this process is incomplete, resulting in **cleft lip and palate**

(Williams, Sandy, Thomas, Sell, & Sterne, 1999). There is no consensus on the cause of this birth defect, but genes and prenatal factors are thought to play a role in disrupting the fusion. (The role of folic acid in birth defects is a promising area of current research.) The majority of the fusion process can be disrupted, resulting in **bilateral complete** clefts of the lip and palate; in other cases, the cleft can be **incomplete** and limited to one side of the oral-maxillary region. Rarely is the cleft limited to the lip. A **submucous cleft** occurs when there is an absence of bone in the palate but the tissue remains intact. In addition, children with cleft lip and palate have a high incidence of middle ear dysfunction and tend to be delayed in language acquisition.

The effect of cleft lip and palate on speech depends on the severity of the defect, the success of surgery in repairing the **orofacial anomalies**, and the results of speech therapy. Three factors ultimately affect speech production in persons with cleft lip and palate. First, cleft lip and related defects of the face can cause articulation disorders, especially of labial phonemes. Usually they interfere only minimally with the child's ability to produce speech because successful surgeries reconstruct the lip and related structures to serve as articulators and therapies teach compensation for residual deficiencies. Second, **nasal emission**, an audible hissing through the nose, can interfere with normal speech production. It is usually a result of **velopharyngeal incompetence**, in which the soft palate does not completely approximate the posterior pharyngeal wall. Not only is the nasal emission obtrusive, it also reduces the amount of air pressure that can be used to produce plosives and other pressure consonants. Third, children with cleft lip and palate can have hypernasality, that is, too much nasal resonance on nonnasal sounds. Hypernasality can result from a slow, sluggish velum or an unrepaired cleft. The speech-language pathologist is a key member of the cleft palate team and addresses the communication disorders associated with this birth defect.

Vocal Cord Paralysis

The vocal cords can be paralyzed by strokes, tumors, degenerative neurological and muscular diseases, and trauma. The **paralysis** or **paresis** (weakness) may involve abduction or adduction of one or both sides of the vocal folds. Spastic paralysis of the larynx results from bilateral upper motor neuron damage. Duffy (1995) has identified unilateral upper motor neuron dysarthria that can affect phonation. It results in weakness on the opposite side of the body and resulting **dysphonia** (impaired voice; **aphonia**: loss of voice). Spastic vocal cord paralysis is common in strokes, reducing the range of motion of the vocal cords. Spastic laryngeal paralysis often causes a harsh or hoarse voice quality. When the cerebellum and the tracts leading to and from the larynx are damaged, ataxia occurs in which vocal movements are poorly coordinated. "Whether or not dysphonia is present may depend upon the severity of the ataxia. The dysphonia may take one of several forms: sudden bursts of loudness, irregular increases in pitch and loudness or coarse voice tremor" (Aronson, 1990, p. 100). Flaccid dysphonia results from damage to cranial nerve X. Usually in flaccid vocal cord paralysis, the voice quality is breathy. In addition, damage at various levels of the neurological system causes laryngeal tremors, uncontrolled jerks, spasms, and voice arrest. The treatment for laryngeal paralysis depends on the type of paralytic dysfunction and may include exercises for forcing the unimpaired vocal cord across the midline, improving range of motion, and strengthening laryngeal muscles. Voice quality, loudness, and pitch modulation are also addressed.

Cancer of the Larynx

Laryngeal growths can be **benign** or **malignant**. Benign growths are **nodules** or **polyps** resulting from vocal strain and abuse (see the section Voice Disorders Related to Vocal Strain and Abuse). Malignant (cancerous) growths tend to worsen if not destroyed by chemical or radiation therapy or surgically removed. Malignant growths also destroy other tissue and can **metastasize**, or spread, to other parts of the body. Decades of research have linked cigarette smoking and the use of other tobacco products to oral and laryngeal cancer.

Improved radiation therapy and chemotherapy for laryngeal cancer have reduced, but not eliminated, the necessity for **complete laryngectomy**, the removal of the entire larynx. In addition, metastasis of the cancer to adjacent tissue may require a radical neck dissection, involving removal of lymph nodes and other tissue. **Partial laryngectomy** involves removal of one vocal cord or part of it. Laryngectomies are extremely disfiguring surgeries, and loss of voice is a major quality-of-life consideration many patients must face. In fact, MacNeil, Weischselbaum, and Pauker (1981), in a study of laryngeal cancer and treatment options, found that most subjects would be willing to reduce their life expectancy to retain the ability to speak. Byrne, Walsh, Farrelly, and O'Driscoll (1993) found an association between depression and poor communication skills in laryngectomized patients.

There are three methods of **alaryngeal speech**. First, a **pneumatic device** can direct the air through the speech mechanism by plugging the **stoma** (an opening through the neck). Second, the patient with a laryngectomy can use an electronic larynx (**electrolarynx**) which provides a vibrating source placed on the patient's neck; the energy is directed upward through the oral and nasal cavities, and the patient "mouths" the words. Third, **esophageal speech**, or *belch talking,* allows the patient to produce near-normal speech by partially swallowing a small amount of air and talking while gradually expelling it. Depending on the patient's capabilities and preferences, the above methods can be used to produce speech in patients with laryngectomies. Some patients prefer to write and gesture rather than to learn these methods.

Other Diseases Affecting the Voice

In **progressive neuromuscular disorders**, the first indication of the disorder may consist of speech difficulties, particularly laryngeal functioning. Patients report unusual pitch changes, vocal tremor, voice quality aberrations, difficulty controlling loudness, and so forth. As the disorder progresses, these symptoms often increase in frequency and severity. Many diseases can cause dysphonia or aphonia. Rather than listing the many diseases affecting laryngeal functioning, it is convenient to categorize them relative to the damaged neurological pathways (Aronson, 1990; Darley, Aronson, & Brown, 1975). Damage to the cerebellum, extrapyramidal system, and upper and lower motor neurons can cause clusters of voice symptoms unique to each neurological level.

Diseases affecting the cerebellum can result in ataxic dysphonia but usually do not cause changes in the vocal cords that can be observed on visual inspection as noted previously, because the cerebellum regulates and coordinates fine motor movements, pitch, loudness, and voice quality changes may be heard. Extrapyramidal dysphonias may be quick or slow. According to Aronson (1990), quick, jerky, irregular, and unpredictable laryngeal movements can be caused by damage to the basal ganglia. These unwanted movements result in sudden forced inspiration or expiration, excess volume variations, and voice quality changes. Dystonia and athetosis are slower forms of hyperkinesia and result in pitch, loudness, phrasing, and voice quality disorders. (Prolonged use of medication can cause tardive dyskinesia and resulting dysphonia.) Parkinson's disease, resulting from damage to the extrapyramidal system and a reduction in the neurotransmitter dopamine, causes hypokinetic dysarthria with slow, unwanted laryngeal movements. Patients with Parkinson's disease often have laryngeal tremor, reduced volume, and monopitch. Upper (pseudobulbar) and lower (bulbar) motor neuron damage can result in spastic and flaccid vocal cord functioning, respectively. Typically, spastic dysphonia results in a harsh voice, with restricted pitch and loudness, and flaccid dysphonia in a breathy voice quality. Voice therapy for the above diseases depends on the type of dysfunction and may include behavioral management, counseling, and instruction to reduce unwanted movements, improving the strength and tone of muscles, and exercises to improve loudness, voice quality, and pitch modulation.

Voice Disorders Related to Vocal Strain and Abuse

Vocal nodules, polyps, and **contact ulcers** are the primary voice disorders related to **vocal strain and abuse**. The list of **vocally abusive behaviors** is long and includes talking too loudly and too much, speaking at a suboptimal pitch, hard glottal attacks, frequent and abusive throat clearing, abusive singing, and others. Exposure to irritating chemical fumes, acid reflux, the use of cigarettes and other tobacco products, and excessive use of alcohol also can be vocally abusive. As discussed at the beginning of this chapter, the vocal cords vibrate very rapidly, and even a small amount of vocally abusive behavior can result in vocal nodules, polyps, and contact ulcers. These growths usually occur on the vocal cord opposite the dominant hand and at the juncture of the anterior and middle commissures of the vocal process, the point of maximal contact force during most phonation.

Vocal nodules, benign tumors about the size of a peppercorn, can occur on either or both vocal cords. They are more common in women and are sometimes called *teachers', preachers',* and *singers' nodes.* Female teachers tend to have voice problems more frequently than male teachers (Smith, Kirchner, Taylor, Hoffman, & Lemke, 1998), and teaching effectiveness is linked directly to the use of the voice (Schmidt, Andrews, & McCutcheon, 1998). A vocal polyp is a fluid-filled blister that may be **sessile** (broad-based) or **pedunculated** (hanging down from a stem). Some physicians consider vocal polyps and **prenodules** to be precancerous. A contact ulcer is an abrasion of the vocal cords. It is more common in men than in women, and the ulceration may be **granulated**. A granuloma is a firm, persistent, inflammatory lesion (Dirckx, 2001).

The goal of treating voice disorders resulting from vocal strain and abuse is to eliminate or minimize the vocally abusive habits. For patients with gaps between their habitual and optimal pitch, behavior modification, instruction, and counseling can be used to help them use their optimal pitch habitually. These methods can also be used to reduce the frequency and severity of hard glottal attacks, abusive throat clearing, and loud, excessive speaking. For singers, instruction and training by professional coaches may be required. Ending the patient's exposure to irritating chemicals and providing medical management of acid reflux also may be warranted, particularly for those with contact ulcers. It is desirable, but often difficult, to have patients stop using tobacco products and alcohol. Teaching the patient to speak with more relaxed laryngeal muscles also helps to reduce vocal fold contact pressure (Tanner, 1991, 2003c).

Psychogenic Voice Disorders

Aronson (1990) lists several **psychogenic voice disorders** including musculoskeletal tension impairments, mutational falsetto, and childlike speech in adults. Musculoskeletal tension disorders are a result of environmental stress. Patients may have a foreign body sensation in the throat, difficulty swallowing, voice quality changes, and aphonia. Mutational falsetto, also known as *puberphonia,* is the failure to change from the higher-pitched voice of the preadolescent to the lower-pitched voice of the adult. "This high-pitched falsetto type is weak, thin, breathy, hoarse, and monopitched, giving the overall impression of immaturity, effeminacy, and passiveness" (Aronson, 1990, p. 136). Childlike speech and voice patterns in adults may result from psychological regression—the retreat to an earlier, more comfortable psychological state due to stress. Childlike speech relieves the person of the responsibility of relating to others in an adult manner.

Hysterical aphonia and dysphonia are common psychogenic voice disorders. They are considered a result of a **conversion reaction** in which the person loses the voice because of psychic trauma related to environmental stress or interpersonal conflicts. Some voice specialists have proposed that the loss of voice **symbolizes** impaired, diminished, or absent communication with significant others. Persons with hysterical aphonia or dysphonia may be involved in unsatisfying or dangerous interpersonal relationships. Some of them seem to welcome the disorder and demonstrate indifference or relief. In the psychiatric literature, this reaction is called **la belle indifference** (in French, "the beautiful indifference"). Hysterical aphonia and dysphonia must be treated by a mental health professional who is trained to deal with the patient's underlying psychological and social dysfunctions. According to Ramig and Verdolini (1998), clinical and experimental data support the effectiveness of therapy for the treatment of psychogenic voice disorders.

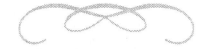

Case Studies in Voice and Resonance Disorders

Case Study 4.1   A 54-Year-Old Man with a Complete Laryngectomy

TIM KNOTT

Tim Knott survived the Vietnam War and retired from the military as a two-star general. He had lived through many stressful nighttime aircraft carrier landings and had survived hundreds of sorties and ground-to-air missile attacks. He had also survived a colossal mixup in which, short of fuel and flying on fumes, he could not find the refueling air tanker. Tim had even weathered a horrendous explosion of bombs and missiles on an aircraft carrier's flight deck. But tragically, he could not prevail over the damage caused by cigarettes. He succumbed to throat cancer after years of battling the disease that took his voice and eventually his life.

Tim requested a voice evaluation from a private speech and hearing clinic after having a hoarse voice for nearly 6 months. He also complained of a foreign body sensation in his throat. The initial evaluation confirmed the hoarse voice quality, and as per standard protocol, he was told to seek a medical examination; otherwise, no voice therapy would be provided. This was particularly important in Tim's case because he was over age 50 and a heavy smoker. He scheduled an appointment with a local otolaryngologist.

The otolaryngologist did a comprehensive laryngeal evaluation and, as was usual at that time, conducted an indirect laryngoscopy. Tim sat in a chair with a light source behind him. The bright light was directed over his shoulder onto an eye mirror on the doctor's head. This mirror has a small hole in it allowing the doctor to direct the reflected light to a dental mirror placed at the back of Tim's throat. The dental mirror reflected the light source down the throat, revealing the vocal cords. The doctor pushed a tongue blade down on Tim's tongue to maximize the viewing surfaces. He saw two small growths on the vocal cords and decided to remove them surgically.

On the morning of surgery, Tim was given a general anesthetic. A scope with a device to cut the growths from his vocal cords was lowered down his throat. Once the nodules were removed, they were sent to the hospital's lab for biopsy. Within hours, the results were available; the nodules were benign. However, many months later, Tim was diagnosed with cancer of the larynx. There were several possible reasons why it had not been discovered during the earlier surgery. Either the cancer had not yet developed, the biopsies were wrong (false negatives), or the cancer was below the vocal cords and out of sight during the laryngoscopy and surgery. Sadly, had the cancer been discovered earlier, perhaps a complete laryngectomy and radical neck dissection would have not been required. By the time the cancer was discovered, it had spread beyond the larynx to adjacent tissue. Consequently, Tim's entire larynx was removed, along with some tissue in his neck and shoulder. He also endured radiation therapy and chemotherapy.

Clinical Sidebar 4.1
Surgical removal of the larynx is called *laryngectomy.* Sometimes a person who has had this surgery is called a *laryngectomee.* Although this term is commonly used, it is not courteous. A person should not be referred to as a communication disorder, but instead should be called *a person with a laryngectomy.* Can you think of other medical situations in which the person is referred to as a disease or disorder?

Between the time of nodule surgery and the diagnosis of cancer, Tim received voice therapy. The therapy was provided to prevent the return of the nodules in the mistaken belief that they were a result of vocal strain and abuse. Initially, Tim's voice improved but the hoarseness was not eliminated. The voice therapy was ultimately unsuccessful, Tim's voice degenerated, he became aphonic, and the laryngectomy was performed.

After the laryngectomy, Tim chose to use an electrolarynx rather than other alaryngeal methods of communicating. He purchased a high quality vibrator from a telephone company and quickly learned how to use it. At first, its use was painful because his neck was sore due to the surgery and radiation treatments. Gradually, he was able to tolerate more pressure on his upper neck. Tim learned that by firmly placing the vibrating diaphragm of the electrolarynx on his neck and directing the energy upward through his oral and nasal cavities, he could produce intelligible, clear speech by mouthing the sounds. The electrolarynx creates a buzzing, "metallic" type of speech, but it is usually intelligible. In addition, the type of electrolarynx used by Tim had a variable frequency setting so that he could adjust the vibration of the diaphragm to maximize the efficiency and quality of his artificial voice. The off-on button was used to produce sound only during the actual utterance, reducing the obtrusiveness of his speech.

Even after the laryngectomy and the news that the cancer had returned and spread, Tim remained active and upbeat. He could no longer pilot his private single-engine Piper Cub airplane due to his communication disorder and because one hand had to hold the electrolarynx in place while talking. However, his friends with private pilot licenses frequently took him on pleasure flights where he could again take the controls, execute steep dives, make hard banks, and soar over the mountains and lakes of the country he had served so well.

Case Study 4.2 A 24-Year-Old Man with Unilateral Adductor Paralysis

BRYAN

Bryan graduated from the university with a degree in civil engineering. In college, he had worked evenings as a bartender but still had thousands of dollars in student loans. Finally, after 5 grueling years, his hard work paid off. Bryan got his first job as a civil engineer and began surveying an addition to the interstate highway system. Years later, Bryan would start his own engineering company, which would become one of the largest in the state. However, throughout his life, he would be plagued by the inability to speak loudly—a constant source of irritation because it interfered with his ability to communicate at job sites. Bryan's vocal cords had been damaged in a terrible car accident during the second week of his first job.

Bryan and two surveyors were returning from the site of the new overpass. The cloverleaf interchange would provide safe access to the freeway for thousands of motorists. The evening sun was just starting to disappear below the high desert horizon as they drove their jeep onto the freeway. The surveyors were sitting in the front of the vehicle and Bryan was in the back seat. Unexpectedly, a sedan with an intoxicated driver hit the rear of the jeep. Later, the Highway Patrol investigators concluded that this driver was traveling at nearly 100 miles per hour, and the sun had blocked his vision. He and the two surveyors were killed. Bryan was propelled forward, his larynx crushed by the metal bar on the front seat of the jeep, and as the jeep rolled into the gutter, he was thrown onto the freeway.

Bryan would have died that summer evening had it not been for a good samaritan. The police investigators suspected that the person who did the emergency tracheotomy was either an off-duty emergency medical technician or a nurse. When Bryan's larynx was crushed, he was unable to breathe. The motorist saw Bryan's respiratory distress, cut a small hole in his neck just below the larynx, and placed a tube in the hole for breathing. The tube was the casing of a pen. When the ambulance arrived, the motorist melted into the crowd of spectators and was never found. The doctors in the hospital's intensive care unit believed that the emergency tracheotomy was too meticulous to have been done by a lay person but not professional enough to have been done by a surgeon. Regardless of the surgical competence, that anonymous motorist had saved Bryan's life. Bryan endured several surgeries to repair his larynx. Ultimately, normal structure and function were restored except for muscular movement on the right side. The laryngeal nerve had been severed, leaving Bryan's vocal cord paralyzed on one side, a condition called *unilateral adductor paralysis.*

The State Vocational Rehabilitation Department's counselor arranged for Bryan's rehabilitation. Because the accident had occurred during work, he was covered by the rehabilitation program. The rehabilitation counselor worked with professionals from several disciplines to help Bryan return to gainful employment. He received occupational and physical therapy for his broken pelvis, hand, and arm and counseling to deal with the anger and grief resulting from the accident. Bryan also received therapy for the unilateral adductor paralysis, which ultimately helped to restore his voice.

At first, Bryan could not produce any vocal cord vibration. All that he could manage was a loud whisper. The clinician showed him that doing strenuous exercises while trying to produce a voice would force the unimpaired vocal cord to contact the paralyzed one. The strenuous exercises and grunting did produce some voice. The clinician had Bryan do pushups, situps, and pull-ups while shouting sounds, syllables, and words. Isometric exercises, in which he pulled or pushed on a body part, also resulted in the necessary muscular force to produce a voice. Bryan jokingly called the voice therapy "boot camp." Gradually his voice improved, and eventually he could voice during normal conversation. Of course, because there was only one vocal cord with functional movement, his voice had a low-pitched, breathy-hoarse quality, and he was able to talk loudly only with great effort. After several months of therapy, the quality of his voice was the best that could be achieved. Bryan was then scheduled to see a laryngologist about a vocal fold implant.

Clinical Sidebar 4.2
In some patients with unilateral adductor paralysis, a physician may be able to inject a solution into the paralyzed vocal fold. This will allow the paralyzed vocal cord to be closer to the midline, increasing the ability of the nonparalyzed vocal fold to approximate it. However, physicians are usually reluctant to do this procedure if the patient has compromised respiration. Can you name several diseases that compromise respiration?

The goal of this implant is to increase the size of the paralyzed vocal cord and move it closer to the midline so that the normal vocal cord has less distance to travel to approximate it. It was hoped that this procedure would increase the loudness and improve the quality of Bryan's voice. The laryngologist first injected a solution into the vocal cord that eventually would be absorbed by his system. This was done to determine the amount of permanent solution that would be necessary to achieve the best voice quality. Later, the correct amount of the permanent solution was injected into the paralyzed vocal fold. This procedure significantly improved Bryan's voice. His conversational and shouted loudness increased by several decibels, and his voice quality improved. Several more voice therapy sessions were conducted to maximize the results of the medical procedure.

Bryan was discharged from voice therapy with near-normal voice quality. Although his habitual pitch was lower than before and his vocal quality was hoarse, Bryan's ability to talk was socially and vocationally functional, except for his inability to talk loudly at job sites. However, persons meeting Bryan for the first time sometimes asked if he had a cold, never suspecting that his voice quality was the result of a terrible motor vehicle accident.

Case Study 4.3 A 23-Year-Old Preacher with Vocal Nodules

JOSEPH

Joseph was the youngest person in the small but growing fundamentalist church to ever have his own congregation. He was just 22 years old when his minister father died, and Joseph was the natural choice to replace him since he had been the youth minister for several years. Joseph had never questioned his religion, as did some of his boyhood friends, and he knew from a young age that the ministry was his calling.

Joseph's father had groomed his only son to follow in his footsteps. When Joseph was very young, he traveled throughout the Midwest with his father to revivals, which were usually held in huge tents on the outskirts of small towns. They were well attended by the faithful, and Joseph admired his father's preaching skills.

He had the power to bring the audience to a frenzy, usually culminating in the "rebirth" of several men and women. As a result of the revival, many persons whose lives had lost meaning took a different road and, in Joseph's eyes, a better one.

In junior high school, Joseph took several church jobs and soon people saw his special gift. Many believed he had a God-given power of speech. Even as a teenager the church was packed during his guest sermons. Later, when he became the youth minister, the young people of the church marveled at his command of the language and his ability to bring God into their lives. He even appeared to have been blessed as a faith healer.

When Joseph was ministering, he lost himself in the power of God. He never paused to search for the correct words. They just seemed to appear in his mind; each word was said clearly and emphatically. The sermons flowed from his lips with grace and ease, and he had a powerful voice. He emphasized important ideas by prolonging vowels and making the first and last syllables of words louder. Joseph never needed a microphone. His booming, low-pitched, resonant voice reached the back of the church, and even those on the sidewalk could hear his words. Sometimes Joseph was so caught up in the message of God that he broke into "tongues," uttering words having meaning only to him and God. All who knew Joseph suspected that someday he would become a televangelist and preach to the world. However, two persistent small growths on his vocal cords derailed his meteoric climb in the world of evangelism.

Clinical Sidebar 4.3
Some patients who develop vocal nodules, polyps, and contact ulcers may say that their voice disorders are not related to vocal strain and abuse. They may report that they have "always talked that way" and question why the voice disorder developed later in life. The disorder may be related to the fact that, as persons age, their laryngeal structures and tissue change, becoming more vulnerable to damage. What anatomical and physiological changes are associated with aging?

The first indication that all was not well with Joseph's voice was fatigue. Soon after he took over the congregation, he noticed that his voice gave out toward the latter part of the services. His booming sermon gradually disintegrated into a whisper. There was also a soreness in his throat and a feeling that something foreign had lodged there, causing frequent throat clearing. The frustration he felt was overwhelming, and he suspected that evil forces were at work to prevent him from spreading the word of God. That frustration took him to a laryngologist, who discovered nodules on his vocal cords, and performed surgery to remove them. For a short time after the surgery, his voice returned to normal. However, like a plague, the communication disorder returned. The laryngologist explained that vocal nodules were not the disorder. They were a symptom of vocal strain and abuse; for a permanent cure, Joseph needed voice therapy.

During the first meeting with the clinician, Joseph was counseled about the nature of therapy for vocal nodules. He learned that there is a curative phase in which the speech behaviors causing and perpetuating the nodules are eliminated. During this phase, Joseph would need to make a serious commitment to change his speech patterns. After the curative phase ended, Joseph would need to adopt certain lifelong speech habits to prevent the nodules from recurring. He would also learn the early signs of vocal nodules so that he could take preventive measure at the first stages of their development.

The clinician explained that the growths on Joseph's vocal folds, sometimes called *preacher's nodes,* had resulted from forcing his voice. Although Joseph used several abusive behaviors in conversational speech, the clinician believed that the sermons were the main culprits. Together, they reviewed several audiotapes of his sermons and identified the abusive speech patterns.

One of the most abusive aspects of Joseph's sermons was their sheer loudness. The clinician explained that loudness is a result of forcing the vocal cords together with great force. The harder the vocal cords come together, the louder the voice. Joseph habitually shouted his sermons. He and the clinician agreed that this aspect of the problem could be solved by using the church's public address system.

Joseph had also gotten into the habit of frequently clearing his throat. This was understandable; the irritation on his vocal cords signaled the presence of foreign bodies. The natural response was to remove them, hence the constant throat clearing. However, clearing the throat is an abusive practice that further irritated his vocal cords, causing further throat clearing—a vicious circle. To stop this self-defeating behavior, Joseph learned to carry water and to drink it whenever he felt the throat irritation. He also learned to clear his throat easily and gently, with the least amount of vocal abuse.

Another vocally abusive behavior was Joseph's speech delivery. His sermons were punctuated with hard glottal attacks in which he emphasized the first words of sentences with increased loudness and extreme pitch variations. Joseph feared that reducing this practice would render his sermons boring and monotonous. However, he also realized that unless he changed his speaking style, his days as a minister were numbered. Joseph and the clinician agreed that a compromise was necessary.

The compromise involved the emphasis Joseph placed on sounds, syllables, and words during his sermons. At one extreme, Joseph could continue to use his previous strong increases in loudness and abrupt changes in pitch to dramatize his speech. This type of delivery would cause chronic voice problems and possibly permanent damage to his voice. At the other extreme, Joseph could deliver his sermons with monoloudness and monopitch, using softly spoken words and phrases. That delivery was unacceptable to Joseph, who feared it would create boring and uninspiring church services. The compromise involved minimizing the vocally abusive behaviors, using the public address system, speaking with relaxed speech musculature, bathing the vocal cords in plenty of liquids, and resting the voice before and immediately after the sermons. To achieve this compromise, during several therapy sessions Joseph practiced his delivery to learn the strategies of reducing the vocal abuse.

Although the compromise did not completely eliminate Joseph's chronic voice disorder, it reduced its frequency and severity. Joseph no longer required surgery, and his voice did not fade to a whisper at the end of the services. He continued the ministry and learned to deal with his voice disorder and the propensity to develop vocal nodules. Joseph viewed the disorder as a test of his faith and resolve as an evangelist.

Case Study 4.4   A 22-Year-Old Woman with Psychogenic Aphonia

BETSY

It seemed that Betsy had always been at odds with her mother. Both women were intelligent and strong-willed, and they frequently clashed. While growing up, Betsy had had a close relationship with her father, but after her parents' divorce, he moved to the West Coast. Betsy spent several summers with him, but during the school year their relationship was limited to weekly telephone calls. After graduating from high school, Betsy took several low-paying jobs that required her to live at home. When she turned 21, she became a bartender at a tavern frequented by college students. Shortly afterward, Betsy lost her voice.

Betsy could not identify the source of stress between her and her mother. In high school, their clashes had occurred over her choice of boyfriends, driving the family car, tattoos, clothing, and keeping her room clean. Betsy felt that she could not rationally discuss anything about her life with her mother. Her mother would automatically react with anger and disapproval, refuse to allow her to drive, take away her pitiful allowance, or give her the silent treatment. The war between them lasted throughout high school. As a young woman, Betsy wanted to discuss her fears, hopes, disappointments, and dreams, but her mother did not seem to have the time or the inclination. Betsy knew that being a single mother, working full time, and having menopausal sleepless nights and hot flashes were hard for her mother, but she was disappointed by her mother's apparent lack of interest and negative attitude. Betsy's friends said that all mother-daughter relationships were trying, but she suspected that the lack of meaningful communication between herself and her mother was extreme.

At work, Betsy and a coworker began a relationship. As usual, her mother disapproved and asked why she could not date someone with a better future. Betsy was amused by mother's idea that young people still dated and that modern women considered men's future earning power as a factor in the mating equation. To Betsy, on those rare occasions when her mother broached an important subject like this relationship, she showed just how little she cared and how far removed from young people's lives she had become. To make matters worse, Betsy's new relationship was not going well and in fact was becoming dangerous. The man was very possessive and had become abusive. He had yet to harm her physically, but it was clear that he was not averse to controlling her in that way. Sex was also becoming frightening; he was no longer gentle and considerate. Sex was becoming another way of exercising control over her. Betsy ached to talk to someone about the direction of her life.

Betsy tried talking to her father, but she could not bring herself to discuss important life issues by telephone; she also wondered if he would understand. She often tried to discuss the relationship with her mother, but each time her mother automatically assumed the worst and reminded Betsy that she had "told her so." Their conversations were one-sided and unsatisfying. Her mother did not understand, and to Betsy, it seemed that she did not want to spend the time and energy needed to understand. Betsy tried talking to her best friend, but since she had recently married, their friendship had suffered. There was no one in Betsy's life who seemed to care enough or to take the time to talk to her. She felt completely alone and did not know how to deal with her problem.

After an argument with her boyfriend, Betsy lost her voice. There was shouting and crying, and he threatened to harm her if she continued to be friendly to customers. At some level, Betsy knew that her loss of voice was not real and that she was capable of vibrating her vocal cords. However, she refused to consciously acknowledge the psychogenic nature of her aphonia. In fact, she was indifferent to the loss of her voice and somehow considered it a blessing. The aphonia had lasted for nearly 2 weeks when her mother suggested that Betsy see a laryngologist. It was the first real gesture of concern she had shown. The laryngologist completed an evaluation and referred Betsy to a speech-language pathologist. Subconsciously, Betsy welcomed the attention.

Clinical Sidebar 4.4
Psychogenic aphonia can be discerned by having the patient hum, laugh, or cough. Because there is no physical cause for the loss of voice, the patient may produce phonation when performing these actions. However, when speaking, he or she will whisper. Have you ever seen something that was so startling that you temporarily lost your speech?

The speech-language pathologist conducted several tests and examinations. Betsy was asked to say sounds, syllables, words, and phrases. She was encouraged to produce a voice by simply trying harder, saying sounds with her chin elevated, and speaking with a lot of air in her lungs. The clinician also tried to get Betsy to laugh; several jokes were told, and she laughed freely. The clinician asked Betsy to hum the tune "Row, Row, Row Your Boat," and she complied without giving it a second thought. Afterward, the clinician showed her how to prolong the sounds of the tune and then to talk the same way. She merged humming into speech. It was like a miracle; Betsy could vibrate her vocal cords during speech. During the remainder of the session, she hummed sounds, words, and phrases. It was easy to turn humming into voiced speech, and by the end of the session Betsy was talking normally. Then the speech-language pathologist said that Betsy should see a psychiatrist. She was told that her loss of voice was a signal that all was not well in her life and that her voice disorder might symbolize lack of communication.

Betsy told the clinician about her mother and her boyfriend. The clinician called the local mental health clinic and arranged an appointment. The clinician was aware of Betsy's financial situation and knew that the clinic offered services on a sliding fee scale.

The meeting with the psychiatrist was short but helpful. The clinician prescribed an antidepressant for Betsy and arranged for counseling through the clinic. The antidepressant would have to be taken for about 6 months, and longer if warranted. Individual and group therapy sessions would last until Betsy felt they were no longer necessary. She learned that she was clinically depressed and probably had been for many years. In therapy, Betsy discovered that she had an immature relationship with her mother and was encouraged to get her own apartment, which she did. She found roommates with positive lifestyles, jobs, and healthy relationships. She learned to separate her feelings about her mother from what her mother said and did. By separating the person from the behaviors, Betsy was free to feel anger at her mother, which apparently she had been suppressing and repressing. Betsy immediately stopped seeing her boyfriend but broke off the relationship carefully, in a way that would not place her in danger. In therapy, Betsy learned a lot about relationships and eventually became an independent woman capable of managing her life. In many ways, Betsy's emotional growth was precipitated by her loss of voice and the professionals who treated it.

Case Study 4.5   Litigation Involving Laryngeal Tissue Scarring from a Kiln Accident

KENDRA

The university and the Board of Regents, the defendants, took the position that Kendra was lying or, at the very least, exaggerating her symptoms. Kendra and her family, the plaintiffs, alleged that her loss of voice and related respiratory conditions were real and possibly fatal. The defendants held that Kendra had violated university regulations when she entered the Fine Arts Building on a Saturday and, without supervision, began her pottery assignment. Kendra and her family stated that she, as a teaching assistant, was issued a building and room key, and that it was implied that she had unlimited access to the kiln and other facilities. The defendants denied liability in the accident because Kendra, a graduate student, should have known that the sawdust she used was not treated to prevent the flash fire. The plaintiffs said that the untreated wood was an attractive nuisance and that the defendants had failed to exercise proper care by not locking it in a secure place, away from students. The defendants proposed that Kendra was faking and that her attempt at deception about her voice disorder was typical of her case. More than $1 million in medical bills, compensation, and damages for pain and suffering were at stake, and the case eventually became a nasty battle of expert witnesses.

The flash fire had taken Kendra by surprise. She had pulled the ceramic pot from the kiln and poured a bucket of sawdust on it, a method used to cool pots to give them a better appearance. This particular batch of sawdust was not treated with a special fire retardant to prevent it from bursting into flames. When the flash fire happened, Kendra had reflexively gasped, inhaling the hot fumes and allegedly suffering burns to her respiratory tract. The types of respiratory burns she had suffered are not uncommon in firefighters, and tragically, they can be fatal. In Kendra's case, allegedly there was progressive scarring of the sensitive lung tissue. After she was released from the burn unit of the hospital, she required supplemental oxygen provided by a small blue tube with holes venting it into her nose. She carried the oxygen bottle everywhere she went. Without it, Kendra could barely walk from her car to the outpatient waiting room at the hospital. She also complained of light-headedness since the kiln accident. This fit young woman, who had previously run marathons, had gained nearly 40 pounds, largely due to her inability to exercise and, according to the doctors, because of the steroids and other medications required to prevent further damage to her lungs.

At the trial, the defendants' expert witness stated that Kendra was exaggerating her symptoms and faking her voice disorder to increase the damages the jury might award her. The expert suggested that although there was likely damage to her lungs, she still could exhale enough air to vibrate her vocal cords. He pointed out that persons with severe chronic obstructive pulmonary diseases, in which the functional volume of air inhaled and exhaled is reduced, are still able to produce a voice. In the expert's opinion, there was no physiological reason for Kendra's inability to produce a voice and the condition was possibly psychogenic. During cross-examination, his credentials were examined and he was questioned about how he had reached this conclusion.

Clinical Sidebar 4.5

Malingering is the willful and deliberate feigning or exaggerating of an illness or disorder for a self-serving end. The purpose is usually financial but can also include exemption, attention, sympathy, and academic and employment rewards. The term *functional* is used to refer to a communication disorder that is nonorganic and can include malingering. How can conscious and subconscious malingering be distinguished? Are there levels of awareness in malingering?

The plaintiff's expert witness stated that Kendra's loss of voice was neither an exaggeration of symptoms nor psychogenic. Large, colorful drawings of the respiratory tract and the vocal cords were placed in front of the jury. The plaintiff's attorney led the expert witness through the respiratory and phonatory processes by asking questions about breath support and the myoelastic-aerodynamic factors associated with voice production. She asked the expert witness to take his time and to explain the process in words the jurists and judge would understand.

The plaintiff's expert witness described how the lungs create pressure below the vocal cords to blow them apart. The vocal cords would stay apart if it were not for the elasticity of the muscles in the larynx and air pressure changes that brought them together. The expert demonstrated that little air pressure was necessary to blow apart the vocal cords and create the suction required to bring them together. He put two sheets of paper together and blew between them. Because of the increased velocity of airflow through the constricted part of the sheets, they were sucked together and began to vibrate. According to the expert, this was a demonstration of the Bernoulli principle and an example of how the vocal cords vibrate. The plaintiff's expert said he agreed with the defendant's assertion that Kendra "probably" had enough air support to activate the muscular and aerodynamic forces necessary to vibrate the vocal cords. In litigation, the distinction between *possibly* and *probably* is important.

Conceding that Kendra's breath support was disrupted but was probably enough for the myoelastic-aerodynamic forces to operate, the plaintiff's expert witness explained to the court that a burn, even a minor one, on the sensitive vocal cord tissue could cause loss of voice. The burned vocal cords, combined with the changes in breath support, had probably caused Kendra to lose her voice. The expert explained in detail that if the temperature of the gas was high enough to burn lung tissue, it was likely to be even hotter as it passed through the vocal cords. He opined that even slight scarring of the sensitive tissue would interfere with vocal cord control and feedback. He also explained that in therapy the patient could create occasional voicing when alternating the prephonation and attack stages and stated that, over several months, he had seen no inconsistencies in Kendra's symptoms. Then the plaintiff's witness did what the court expected of him: He gave an educated appraisal of the case and a probable explanation for Kendra's loss of voice. He stated that in his expert opinion, Kendra was neither exaggerating nor faking the disorder.

The trial involved several days of testimony from specialists and others. At the end of the exhausting ordeal, applause and sighs of relief were heard when the jury found for the plaintiff on all counts. Kendra and her family would receive their just compensation for the accident that took her voice and livelihood.

Case Study 4.6 Identical Twins with Cleft Lip and Palate

KYLE AND JAROD

During the ultrasound procedure, the doctor pointed to a vague image and said, "Do you see the head and body?" The prospective parents nodded, although they really could not tell much from the picture on the monitor. Then the doctor said, "Oh, look, there's another one." The startled expectant father sat down on the nearest chair while the doctor continued to discuss the images of the twins. When the doctor left the room, the expectant parents hugged each other and began planning for the two additions to their family. The pregnancy was relatively normal, but during the last few weeks, the woman was required to spend most of her time in bed and take medication to delay premature birth. Early one morning the twins were born, but the joy of their birth was tempered by the sight of their unilateral cleft lips and palates. The obstetrician told the parents that although the cause of this condition would probably never be known, in a certain percentage of cases, it may have a genetic link. In this case, there was a maternal family history of cleft lip and palate; an uncle had been born with the defect. However, it was also possible that during gestation, intrauterine factors may have affected the fetuses and caused the birth defect.

The primary cleft palate team at the Children's Rehabilitation Hospital consisted of a pediatrician, reconstructive surgeon, orthodontist, dental surgeon, audiologist, medical social worker, and speech-language pathologist. Other specialists such as dietitians, nutritionists, and psychologists also participated when necessary. The team met weekly and focused on patients seen in the hospital. The captain was the medical social worker, who organized and conducted the meetings, allowing all team members to present their reports and discuss specific issues. This was the initial meeting with the twins' parents, who were to be members of the team. The first professional to discuss Kyle and Jarod was the pediatrician, who said that she would be the children's primary care doctor until their 18th birthday. She told the parents that children with cleft lip and palate often have special medical needs, and careful monitoring and regular checkups were important. She said that any medical concerns they might have should be addressed to her. She would also arrange and coordinate all intervention activities related to their birth defects.

According to the plastic surgeon, the surgeries to repair the twins' clefts and reconstruct the facial features would begin before their first birthday. He reported that in more than 80% of cases, primary repair of the palate results in adequate velopharyngeal closure. Only a few patients need secondary physical management.

He suspected that because of the nature of their clefts, the twins would likely need secondary management. In addition, the pharyngeal flap surgery, in which tissue is connected between the velum and the posterior pharyngeal wall to aid velar movement and closure, would have to be supplemented by speech therapy.

Clinical Sidebar 4.6

Sometimes surgeons are unable to create velopharyngeal closure in persons with cleft palate. However, there are certain speech behaviors that can minimize nasal emission and hypernasality. For example, altering the patient's habitual pitch may reduce the perception of hypernasality, and teaching the patient to talk with a "more opened" mouth will help direct less airflow and energy through the nose. Why? What aerodynamic principles are at work?

The orthodontist predicted that both children would require extensive orthodontic and dental reconstruction. He and a dental surgeon would do preliminary work on the children's temporary teeth, but the major reconstruction and alignment would be done on the permanent teeth. The orthodontic work would not begin for several years.

The audiologist explained that children with cleft lip and palate have more frequent hearing problems. These problems are primarily middle ear dysfunctions probably caused by eustachian tube abnormalities. The eustachian tube equalizes pressure between the external environment and the middle ear. When this pressure cannot be equalized, earaches and conductive hearing loss can occur. The audiologist also said that tubes could be placed in the eardrums to help equalize the pressure. He concluded that frequent hearing testing was necessary in managing individuals with orofacial anomalies.

The speech-language pathologist indicated that children with cleft lip and palate can have articulation, voice and resonance, and language disorders. Kyle and Jarod might have articulation disorders due to the malformation of their lips, dental processes, and palates. Even after the surgeries, because of the malformations they might have difficulty articulating and receiving sensory information. However, with therapy, this would probably not be a major deterrent to normal articulation. The clinician explained that the surgeries were most important to the children's ultimate ability to speak with proper air pressure and nasality. With good surgical results and therapy, they would likely achieve normal or near-normal speech. Also, according to the clinician, studies show that some children with orofacial anomalies have delayed language development. The delay is probably related to the surgeries, the postsurgical discomfort, and the fact that speech communication is not as rewarding for children with these defects as it is for other children. The clinician concluded by stating that the twins' chances of achieving normal or near-normal communication was very good.

The medical social worker concluded the meeting by discussing the financial costs of the lengthy habilitation process. Few families could pay these costs for even one child, let alone two. The Children's Hospital was funded by several grants and agencies, and most of the costs would be covered by them and by the parents' insurance. The medical social worker explained that she would be a resource for the parents, helping them navigate through the complex habilitation process that would last for many years.

As predicted during the first meeting, Kyle and Jarod underwent several surgeries to repair their clefts. Their palatal shelves, dental processes, and nasal processes were surgically reconstructed, and eventually they appeared normal except for some scarring. Their hearing was regularly tested, and small tubes were placed in their ears. They received speech, voice, and language therapy as hospital outpatients, and they took part in the special education program in elementary school. By the time Kyle and Jarod entered middle school, they were remarkably similar to the other boys in appearance and speech, due largely to the work of the cleft palate team.

Case Study 4.7 Total Laryngectomy in a 66-Year-Old Man with Impeccable Esophageal Speech in Three Sessions

ALVIN THE GREAT

I know that patients with total laryngectomies have contracted laryngeal cancer and have suffered terribly disfiguring surgeries. I appreciate the stress, anxiety, and pain they endure. I have empathy and sympathy for them, but I must confess that I enjoy teaching esophageal speech. For me, there is something rewarding about teaching a patient to shape a belch into speech. Esophageal speech training is challenging, and when you have a patient like Alvin, the product is an amazing communication art form.

For 30 years, Alvin Sharp worked as a janitor in a small school district. He confessed to me that being a janitor was a very rewarding job. He got to work around young people, the hours were reasonable, the pay was acceptable, and most of the time there was no one to boss him around. Alvin knew that being a janitor was not a prestigious position, but for him, that was unimportant; there were many rewarding jobs with little prestige. It didn't take long for me to realize that Alvin was very intelligent. According to a study of persons with high intelligent quotients, many of them take jobs with low stress and great freedom but with low prestige. They prefer to avoid the stress and anxiety of high pressure jobs in business, education, and industry. It struck me that people like Alvin may be smarter than we think.

Alvin came to my speech and hearing clinic at a time when I was questioning my own stress level and rewards. My professional corporation had grown into a large business with several professional employees and office staff, many contracts, and two downtown clinics. My days were spent juggling schedules, reviewing Medicare forms, negotiating contracts, borrowing from IRAs to make payrolls, and dealing with unpleasant issues. Overall, the business was successful, but financially it seemed to be a case of "feast or famine." There was usually too much to do and too little time to do it. When I saw the appointment for a laryngectomy patient, I asked the designated clinician if I could have it, and she agreed. The patient's chart indicated that he had undergone a complete laryngectomy with no complications. He had been counseled presurgically and said that he wanted the esophageal speech option.

The first time I met Alvin, I immediately liked him. He was about 6 feet tall, slender, and completely bald. He had an expressive smile and a strong handshake. To communicate, he wrote a note. Because of the communication barrier, I did most of the talking, explaining the idea behind esophageal speech and showing him several pictures from a textbook. He wrote that he looked forward to being able to talk again and wanted to know how long it would take. I said that individuals learn at different rates and, unfortunately, some patients cannot achieve functional esophageal speech. It would probably take 3 months of individual therapy three times a week, and there would be extensive homework assignments. Recently, a "Lost Chord Club" consisting of persons with laryngectomies had been formed, and I encouraged Alvin to attend the next meeting in 2 weeks. By then, Alvin should be able to say a few words. Then we got down to work, and I explained the injection method.

In my experience, most patients prefer the *piston* injection method, and Alvin was no exception. I showed him how to touch the tongue to the alveolar ridge and capture as much air as possible. Then gradually, using the entire tongue in a progressive movement, I showed Alvin how to move the air mass to the back of the throat, explaining that the air is not swallowed, but held midway in the throat. I demonstrated the process several times and was able to expel an acceptable amount of air. Then I showed Alvin how speech is made on the belching noise coming from that air mass vibrating the lower part of the throat. After several attempts, I could say "I want" with reasonable intelligibility. I explained that the goal is to make a belching sound of sufficient volume and to prolong it as long as possible while mouthing speech. Alvin could probably do better than I did, I observed, because he had more space due to the surgery and fewer structural limitations. Then I asked him to give it a try.

> **Clinical Sidebar 4.7**
> When teaching persons with laryngectomy to use esophageal speech, for some patients it may be more helpful to demonstrate the principles of alaryngeal communication. Once they learn these principles, they may be better able to master speaking using their own techniques rather than following the clinician's step-by-step instructions. Do you learn better by example or by reading instructions?

Alvin carefully touched his tongue to his alveolar ridge and, spreading it out laterally, he gradually pistoned the captured air to the back of his throat and partially down the esophagus. Then, loudly and articulately, he said: "How's that?" Automatically I said, "Fine," before I could register what had just occurred. Believing his utterance was a fluke, I asked him to do it again, and with even more volume and precision, he said, "This is fun." He had actually said the three words on one injection! Thinking that this had to be an episode of *Candid Camera,* I looked around to see if there were any witnesses to this remarkable event. I asked Alvin if he had been getting therapy or practicing before our session, and he said that this was the first time he had tried it since he was a youngster. As a young boy, he and his cousins played games involving belch talking and even had a club where everyone was required to talk that way. He was very proficient, and his skills had not diminished over the years. During the remainder of the session, he continued to show a remarkable esophageal speaking ability. He picked it up so fast that I labeled him "Alvin the Great," a title he appreciated.

We had two more sessions, and by the end of the week I discharged him from therapy. He practiced esophageal speech for several hours each night and by the end of the week had mastered it. I offered advice on improving his intelligibility by exaggerating the precision of articulation and emphasizing sounds in the final positions of words. The only negative speech behavior he acquired was the tendency to produce a "chink" sound during an injection. He was able to eliminate this distracting noise after I brought it to his attention. During the final session, I was treated to his great sense of humor. I was explaining the finer points of coordinating breathing with speaking when he interrupted me, saying, "I'll get a hamburger for lunch." I looked at him quizzically, and he laughingly said, "Sorry about the interruption, but I had a true belch and I didn't want to waste it."

I never saw Alvin again. Several month later, I telephoned him to check on his progress. He said his speech was very good and things were going well. His speech was so good, in fact, that it was difficult to know he had had a laryngectomy; he simply sounded as though he had a cold. Alvin the Great had truly mastered esophageal speech.

SUMMARY

Voice and resonance disorders involve problems with the source of voiced speech sounds, such as occurs with vocal nodules, polyps, and contact ulcers. The most severe sound source-communication disorder is laryngectomy, and patients must learn alternative methods of creating a voice. The sound source may also be impaired when the larynx is damaged or impaired by burns, diseases, traumas, and psychological factors. The voice also involves the resonance occurring in the cavities in the head and neck; orofacial anomalies can cause nasal emission and hypernasality. Most voice disorders are successfully treated with medical and therapeutic management.

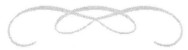

Study and Discussion Questions

1. Compare the workings of a brass or reed musical instrument to the sound source-resonating system of the human voice.

2. Describe the Bernoulli principle and explain how it is partially responsible for closing the vocal cords during phonation.

3. Describe the muscular forces involved in the myoelastic-aerodynamic principle of vocal fold vibration.

4. What are the functions of extrinsic and intrinsic laryngeal muscles?

5. List four voice qualities and discuss the psychological and personality attributes a listener may perceive when hearing them.

6. Describe cleft lip and palate and discuss its likely causes.

7. Discuss the levels of neurological damage and the different types of laryngeal paralysis.

8. What are three methods of alaryngeal speech? Describe them.

9. List vocally abusive behaviors and ways of eliminating or reducing them.

10. Discuss the origins and manifestations of psychogenic voice disorders and ways of obtaining normal speech.

11. List the members of a cleft palate medical team and describe their responsibilities.

12. Describe how you would teach a patient esophageal speech.

Recommended Reading

Aronson, A. E. (1990). *Clinical voice disorders: An interdisciplinary approach* (3rd ed.). New York: Thieme.

This book provides a comprehensive technical examination of voice disorders with case studies and colorful illustrations.

Gobl, C., & Ni' Chasaide, A. (2002). The role of voice quality in communicating emotion, mood and attitude. *Speech Communication, 40* (1–2), 189–212.

This article discusses several voice qualities, emotions, moods, and attitudes.

Ramig, L. O., & Verdolini, K. (1998, February). Treatment efficacy: Voice disorders. *Journal of Speech, Language, and Hearing Research, 41,* S101–S116.

This article presents a comprehensive review of voice therapies and their effectiveness circa 1998.

Tanner, D. (1990). *Tanner muscular relaxation program for voice disorders.* Oceanside, CA: Academic Communication Associates.

This treatment program provides information about reactive voice disorders and their treatment. It includes an instructional cassette tape that helps patients learn to relax their respiratory and laryngeal muscles.

Tanner, D. (2003). *Exploring communication disorders: A 21st century introduction through literature and media.* Boston: Allyn & Bacon.

Chapter 3 of this book uses references to books, films, and media personalities to explore the human voice and its disorders.

Zemlin, W. (1998). *Speech and hearing science* (4th ed.). Boston: Allyn & Bacon.

This is the definitive textbook on the anatomy and physiology of the speech and hearing mechanisms, including vocal functioning.

CHAPTER FIVE

Aphasia

Language most shows a man; speak, that I may see thee.

Ben Johnson

Chapter Preview: In this chapter you will learn about aphasia, a language disorder usually affecting all modalities of communication. There is a discussion of predominantly expressive (nonfluent) and predominantly receptive (fluent) aphasia and the nature of the symptoms. Five psychological concomitants of aphasia are reviewed, and its etiology and rehabilitation are described. There are six case studies addressing traumatically induced jargon aphasia, word-finding problems, telegraphic speech, auditory-acoustic agnosia, aphasia resulting from a brain tumor, and global aphasia. A case study focusing on a rehabilitation team is also presented.

OVERVIEW OF APHASIA AND RELATED DISORDERS

Aphasia is the loss of previously acquired language abilities due to brain damage. It can eliminate the person's ability to speak, read, write, and understand the speech of others. **Dysphasia** is a milder form of the disorder in which the patient retains some ability to use language. Psychologically, aphasia is a double-edged sword. It is caused by serious medical conditions that can create many adjustment challenges and isolate the patient from those who can and want to help. Aphasia can have a devastating effect on the patient's quality of life.

Aphasia has existed presumably since humans began to talk. In the mid-1800s, two neurologists identified parts of the brain important to communication. Paul **Broca**, a French physician, discovered that the left side of the brain controls speech. In 1865, he made this now-famous statement: "We speak with the left hemisphere." Later, a German physician, Karl **Wernicke**, discovered that the left hemisphere is important to understanding speech. Today, the area of the brain important for **expressive** communication is called *Broca's area,* and *Wernicke's area* is its **receptive** counterpart. Together, these sites are considered the major speech and language centers of the brain. Figure 5.1 shows the major speech and language regions of the left hemisphere of the brain found in the majority of (but not all) persons.

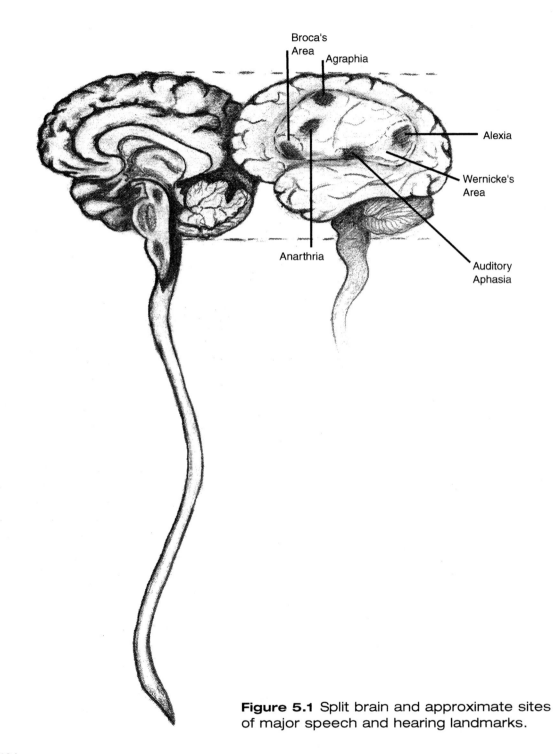

Figure 5.1 Split brain and approximate sites of major speech and hearing landmarks.

Table 5.1 General Classifications of Aphasia

Damage to Broca's and/or Adjacent Areas and Tracts of the Brain	Damage to Wernicke's and/or Adjacent Areas and Tracts of the Brain	Damage to Broca's, Wernicke's, and Adjacent Areas and Tracts of the Brain
Predominantly expressive aphasia	Predominantly receptive aphasia	Severe expressive-receptive aphasia
Motor aphasia	Sensory aphasia	Global aphasia
Nonfluent aphasia	Fluent aphasia	Irreversible aphasia syndrome
Anterior (fissure of Rolando) aphasia	Posterior (fissure of Rolando) aphasia	Complete aphasia
Broca's aphasia	Wernicke's aphasia	Dense aphasia
Telegraphic speech	Jargon aphasia	Profound aphasia

Although certain sites of the brain have been identified as important to expressive and receptive communication, the brain operates as a whole. No part of the brain is completely independent of others. In addition, there is considerable anatomical variation among individuals in the areas for speech and language. In fact, in some persons the left hemisphere is not dominant for language. According to Zemlin (1998) and Restak (1984), the left hemisphere is specialized for language, handedness, analytic thought processes, and certain types of memory in about *90%* of right-handed persons and about *60%* of left-handed persons. In those who are **ambidextrous**, the left hemisphere is dominant in about *60%,* and both brain hemispheres are equally dominant in some. Especially in regard to language, it is difficult to localize one area of the brain as totally responsible for a particular function in all persons.

There are four important factors in understanding aphasia; each is discussed in detail below. First, aphasia is not a **speech impediment**; it is the loss or disruption of language (Darley, 1982; Darley et al., 1975). Second, aphasia impairs to various degrees all **modalities** of language—speaking, gestures, writing, reading, and understanding the words of others. Aphasia also may impair the ability to perform and understand simple mathematics. Third, aphasia can be separated into **predominantly expressive** and **predominantly receptive** disorders. Although aphasia cuts across all modalities of language, most patients have either predominantly expressive or predominantly receptive deficits. Finally, aphasia includes several psychological components, such as excessive emotional reactions, catastrophic reactions (anxiety attacks), and depression. Table 5.1 presents the general classification of aphasia and related disorders.

Etiology of Aphasia

Aphasia can be caused by a wide range of diseases and disorders. **Strokes**, or cerebrovascular accidents, are the most common causes of aphasia. A stroke occurs when parts of the brain are deprived of blood, causing anoxia (lack of oxygen) and the sudden death of tissue (**infarct**). There are two types of strokes: **occlusive** and **hemorrhagic**. An occlusive stroke occurs when an artery supplying blood to the brain is blocked. In one type of occlusive stroke, an **embolus**, an obstruction that originates elsewhere in the body moves and eventually lodges in the brain. By contrast, the occlusive type of stroke known as **thrombosis** develops when the obstruction originates in the brain. A hemorrhage is the rupture of an artery to the brain, with subsequent bleeding and buildup of pressure in the cranial cavity. According to Marquardt (2000, pp. 462–463): "The prevalence and morbidity vary with each of the etiologies of stroke. Thromboses occur more frequently than hemorrhages, but individuals with thrombosis are more likely to survive the stroke." Strokes are the third leading cause of death in the United States (Owens et al., 2000).

Aphasia can also be caused by **traumatic brain injuries**, which can be open or closed. An open traumatic brain injury occurs when a **missile** or **projectile** enters the brain. In a closed head injury, a foreign object does not enter the brain but brain tissue is damaged. Patients with traumatic brain injuries often have reduced awareness, memory loss, and disorientation in addition to neurogenic communication disorders.

Diseases can cause aphasia, the most serious of which is cancer of the brain. A **malignant** brain tumor occupies space, and as it grows, it destroys brain cells. Surgery, radiation treatment, and chemotherapy are used to combat the cancer. Tumors may also be noncancerous (**benign**) but still cause aphasia if they affect the major speech and language centers and the tracts leading to and from them. Virtually any disease or disorder that can damage or destroy the speech and language centers of the brain, and the tracts leading to and from them, can cause aphasia.

Aphasia and Motor Speech Disorders

Apraxia of speech is often a component of aphasia. There are two primary neurogenic communication disorders: aphasia and motor speech disorders. They occur when the ability to communicate is eliminated or impaired due to damage to the brain and/or nervous system. As noted above, aphasia is a language disorder in which semantic processing and grammar can be impaired to varying degrees for both expression and reception. **Semantics** deals with words and their meanings. The word, whether written, gestured, or spoken, is a **symbol**, an arbitrary representation of reality used for communication and thought. The **referent** is that to which the symbol refers. It can be a tangible aspect of reality, such as *chair,* or an abstract concept, such as *truthfulness.* Semantics is the relationship between the symbol and its referent. **Grammar** is the rules by which spoken, written, or gestured language is constructed and understood. It includes rules for combining and sequencing sounds into words and transforming words into sentences and phrases. Aphasia can disrupt or eliminate these previously learned aspects of language. Apraxia of speech and the dysarthrias are the **motor speech disorders**. *Motor* refers to the physical aspects of generating and transmitting a neurological impulse for muscle movement. Motor speech disorders are discussed in Chapter 6.

Aphasia as a Multimodality Disorder

There are several **avenues** or modalities of communication. The linguistic modalities are speaking, listening, writing, and reading. Aphasia impairs, to varying degrees, all modalities of communication. According to Davis (2000), in aphasia "the modalities are not impaired equally, and there is a typical pattern of comparative deficit" (p. 2). The general pattern of aphasic impairment is, from the least to most impaired modality, listening, reading, speaking, and writing. In aphasia, the inability to read is called **alexia**; **dyslexia** is a less severe form of the disorder. **Agraphia** and **dysgraphia** are the inability or impaired ability, respectively, to express oneself using written symbols.

Persons also use **gestural communication**, which has both expressive and receptive modes. They can express themselves using hand, finger, and, to a lesser extent, general body and facial gestures, and the receiver can comprehend them. Aphasia usually impairs the ability to use gestures to express and understand complex thoughts, but basic gestures are preserved in even the most severe aphasia. For example, even a patient with severe aphasia can turn away to express refusal and can appreciate a pat on the back for a job well done. As noted above, aphasia also impairs mathematical abilities; this is because mathematics is also a language. The mathematical disorder is not limited to complex processes such as those of algebra and statistics. It also affects simple problems such as knowing how much change to give, that $2 + 4 = 6$, and how many quarters there are in two dollars. In aphasia, the inability to do and understand simple arithmetic is called **acalculia**; **dyscalculia** is a less severe form of the disorder.

Predominantly Expressive Aphasia

Patients with predominantly expressive aphasia have difficulty **encoding** (formulating) language to express themselves. The **core language deficits** in this form of aphasia are difficulty recalling names and problems in constructing sentences and phrases. There are several types of naming problems in aphasia. Some patients are unable to supply any word for a concept or object. For example, when asked to name objects, they are silent or try to have the listener supply the words. Other patients produce the wrong word and may or may not be aware of the mistake. They may say an incorrect word that is associated with the correct one, such as *pen* for *pencil, knife* for *fork,* or *car* for *truck.* These **association errors** are also called **verbal paraphasias**. Sometimes patients may say words that phonemically approximate or rhyme with the correct word—*fan* for *tan, pen* for *hen,* or *bun* for *run.* These **approximation errors** are also known as **literal paraphasias**. In **random naming errors**, there are no semantic or phonological associations—no rhyme or reason to the word-finding or naming errors. A patient making a random naming error might call a car a banana.

As noted above, predominantly expressive aphasia usually has a motor component. In some instances, the patient can recall the word he or she wants to express but has difficulty programming and sequencing the speech muscles to produce it. The motor aspect of predominantly expressive aphasia involves purposeful speech acts. Usually, there is a **volitional-involitional dichotomy** in programming speech. The patient may be unable to program and sequence the speech muscles for purposeful and voluntary movements but can speak some words automatically and involuntarily.

When aware of the naming error, the patient will often attempt to correct it and may or may not be successful. These attempts to self-correct often render speech **nonfluent**, with hesitations, repetitions, and revisions. Some patients use **tip-of-the-tongue behaviors**, in which production of the word is just out of reach and the patient makes repetitive attempts to say it. Because of their reduced vocabulary and impaired grammar, many patients employ **telegraphic speech**, using content words to the exclusion of grammatical and functional ones. "I bathroom" is a telegraphed utterance indicating that the patient wants to go to the bathroom now.

Predominantly Receptive Aphasia

Patients with predominantly receptive aphasia have problems **understanding** the **writing**, **gestures**, and **speech** of others. They have varying degrees of difficulty **decoding** (analyzing) language. These problems can occur at the **perception** (see the section on Aphasia and Agnosia below) or **association** levels and are more apparent when the amount of information is increased. **Attention deficits** may also be present and may contribute to the decoding impairments. Some patients have **slow rise time**, attending to only the last part of a statement or request. In the opposite reaction, **auditory fade**, the patient attends to only the first part.

Speech in predominantly receptive aphasia is usually **fluent** unless the patient stops to improve self-monitoring. Typically, these patients do not use fluency disruptions such as hesitations, repetitions, and revisions. Many of them also use **jargon speech**, broadly defined as fluent but meaningless utterances, although some aphasia classification systems limit the definition to specific types of utterances. In general, jargon speech can be disrupted by **semantic** or **phonemic factors**. Conventional words may be used in such a way that the sentence has no meaning, such as "It depends on the acrylic, thus far." Jargon speech may also consist of **neologisms** (invented words) such as *kryptocat* or *tula*. Many patients with jargon aphasia produce a combination of made-up words and conventional ones used incorrectly.

Aphasia and Agnosia

Broadly defined, **agnosia** is a **perceptual** disorder in which the patient is unable to recognize salient features of a sensory stimulus. It can be caused by damage to several areas of the brain, especially the **thalamus**, a structure that is sometimes called the **gatekeeper** and is important to perception. Agnosia can affect any of the five senses, but vision and hearing are most relevant to aphasia. Unlike aphasia, which impairs, more or less, all modalities of communication, agnosia is usually limited to one modality. For example, a patient with **visual agnosia** may have difficulty recognizing letters and other graphemes visually, but knows them when they are spoken or traced on his or her hand. In visual agnosia for objects, a patient puts a knife in a glass of water to use it as a straw; visually, he or she does not appreciate the utensil's significance.

Auditory agnosia is impairment of information coming from the sense of hearing, and includes speech and nonspeech stimuli. **Acoustic agnosia** is misperception of the differences in the salient aspects of speech sounds. A patient with auditory agnosia might misperceive the ring of a telephone, a knock at the door, or the high-pitched, steady tone of a smoke alarm—picking up the telephone at the sound of a knock at the door, ignoring a visitor's beckoning at the door, and failing to leave a room when an alarm goes off. In auditory agnosia, the patient misperceives or does not appreciate the significance of environmental sounds. In acoustic agnosia, the auditory discrimination problems are related to speech sounds, with or without environmental sound misperception. Individual speech sounds are not distinguishable, especially those that are acoustically similar. Because it is clinically difficult to diagnose and treat the two disorders separately, in this book perceptual disorders related to the sense of hearing are called *auditory-acoustic agnosia.*

Aphasia and Abstraction

Because language is important to thinking, the question may arise, what role does aphasia play in intelligence? Neuropsychological tests often reveal that the patient with aphasia has a reduced verbal intelligence quotient, but performance scores are usually only moderately reduced or within the normal range. Although aphasia does disrupt or eliminate language, it does not reduce the patient to the mental status of a child, nor does he or she have mental retardation or dementia. Most patients remember life experiences and can process information using nonlanguage modalities. However, it would be misleading to suggest that a patient's cognitive abilities are unaffected by aphasia. Early research on the cognitive abilities of patients with aphasia showed that they tend to use concrete thinking (Goldstein, 1948, 1952). In his classic articles on aphasia and cognition, Goldstein called this condition **abstract-concrete imbalance**. Patients with aphasia tend to function on a concrete level for verbal abilities, as expected, and for nonverbal tasks as well. For example, when sorting tokens of various shapes, colors, and sizes, these patients, particularly those with severe aphasia, tend to be concrete and have problems knowing the categories.

Psychological Concomitants of Aphasia

Although there are individual variations in the way persons react to brain damage, stress, loss, and disability, decades of research have shown common psychological reactions in patients with aphasia. These include catastrophic reactions, perseveration-echolalia, organic depression, a grief response to loss, and emotional lability (Tanner, 2003a, 2003b). Not all patients with aphasia experience all of these reactions, and some, particularly those with mild and reversible aphasia, are spared significant reactions. Many of the psychological concomitants of aphasia are short-lived; others, such as organic depression, may be long-lasting.

The Catastrophic Reaction

The **catastrophic reaction** in aphasia can be viewed as an **anxiety attack**. It is a psychobiological breakdown involving physical changes and negative emotions (Eisenson, 1984). These anxiety attacks can include a variety of behaviors and reactions, including irritability, crying, striking out, withdrawal, and fainting. Patients report a general feeling of uneasiness or a sense of impending doom. A catastrophic reaction can be triggered when too many demands are placed on the patient or when there is too much noise in the immediate environment. It can also occur when the patient is placed in a situation where successful performance is unlikely, threatening his or her sense of self-integrity. Frustration at being unable to complete a task that was once done normally and easily precipitates and perpetuates the catastrophic reaction. Biologically, the fight-or-flight response occurs.

The **fight-or-flight response** is a remnant of human evolution and survival. Early humans confronted with a life-threatening situation had two choices: fight or flee. Today, the fight-or-flight response occurs in life-threatening situations and also in those where the threat is psychological. Confronted with a psychological threat, the person has the biological reactions of fear, anxiety, and panic similar to those accompanying physical threats—increased heart rate, rapid breathing, hypertense muscles, sweating, and elevated blood pressure. According to Laraia (1998), a panic attack occurs when the human alarm system is triggered. Although all patients with aphasia can have catastrophic reactions, these reactions are more common in those with left hemisphere brain damage, particularly in and around Broca's area, and the more nonfluent the speech, the more likely the response (Tanner, 2003a).

Perseveration-Echolalia

Perseveration occurs when the patient is caught in one mental set or behavior pattern and cannot shift easily to another one. The sensory or motor act tends to continue longer than is appropriate or warranted by the stimuli. Observable perseveration occurs during writing and speaking. In graphic perseveration, the patient's writing consists of letters repeated continuously. The hand movements cannot shift from one pattern to another. Often the writing initially appears normal, with the first or second letter produced correctly; then it disintegrates into a flat line. The patient with verbal perseveration uses the same sound, word, or phrase repeatedly. He or she appears to be "locked in," incapable of shifting to another word or concept regardless of what question has been asked. In aphasia, **echolalia**, the automatic repetition of the last word or words spoken by someone else, often occurs with perseveration. Current research suggests that a subcortical structure, the caudate nucleus, is the likely area of damage in perseveration (Kreisler et al., 2000).

Organic Depression

Depression is an emotional disorder characterized by feelings of despair, sadness, reduced self-esteem, and a sense of helplessness and hopelessness. It may be accompanied by anxiety, loss of appetite, sleep disorders, or lethargy. Research shows that as many as *50% to 70%* of patients with aphasia may suffer from chronic **depression-anxiety**. This occurs more frequently in left hemisphere than right hemisphere damage, and the more nonfluent the aphasia, the more likely the patient is to have depression (Tanner, 2003a, 2003b). Many aphasiologists believe that this type of depression is a direct result of the brain injury and of a disruption of neurochemicals that control and regulate mood.

Organic depression is primarily the result of brain chemicals gone awry; it is not reactive, nor is it the kind of depression found in the grief response (see below). Although reactive and grieving factors can contribute to organic depression, this condition is primarily the result of altered brain chemistry because of brain injury or the medications used to treat it.

Response to Loss

Aware patients with irreversible neurogenic communication disorders can experience a multidimensional sense of loss and the reaction to it: the **grief response** (Tanner, 1980, 1999a, 2003a; Tanner & Gerstenberger, 1996). According to Code, Hemsley, and Herrmann (1999), the grief model is powerful due to its ability to explain some of the emotional and psychosocial reactions seen in patients with neurogenic communication disorders, although more research is necessary. Many patients with these disorders experience loss in three dimensions: self, person, and object.

Loss of self occurs when the patient perceives that he or she can no longer function normally. In aphasia, this includes the multimodality inability to communicate and, in many patients, concomitant physical limitations such as difficulty walking. **Loss of person** occurs because the patient is irreversibly separated from loved ones. Although these persons are not physically lost, such as occurs in death, the patient can no longer interact meaningfully with them because of the communication disorder. This psychological separation is compounded by physical separation if the patient is confined to an institution. **Loss of object** occurs when the patient is involuntarily separated from a valued object such as a home, recreational vehicle, or pet. In many aware patients with severe irreversible aphasia, losses of self, person, and object combine to create a great sense of grief and sorrow. Many patients go through several stages in coming to terms with their loss. **Denial**, **anger**, and **bargaining** are attempts to overcome the loss. **Grieving depression** occurs when the patient becomes aware of being irreversibly separated from valued aspects of self, person, and objects. Most patients gradually achieve **acceptance** and **resolution** of their losses. They are not resigned to their fate; they accept it without major negative emotions and activation of psychological defenses.

Emotional Lability

Emotional lability is the tendency toward exaggerated emotions, often associated with bilateral brain damage to the motor strips and associated corticobulbar tracts. The emotional threshold is lowered, and feelings appear to be on the surface. Patients who are emotionally labile often cry too much and too long over apparently little things. They also may laugh too much, but crying is more common. Words, thoughts, and situations may set off bouts of emotional lability, and once begun, they are difficult for the patient to control.

In the past, emotional lability was considered an inappropriate response or one with no true emotions, just the behavior of crying (or laughing) devoid of feeling. We now know that these emotional responses are not inappropriate; they are exaggerated. The patients' affect and feelings associated with the neurogenic communication disorder and related disabilities are appropriate but excessive.

Treatment of Aphasia

Many patients with aphasia make a **spontaneous recovery**, regaining their communication abilities without the benefit of treatment. The rate of improvement is greatest soon after aphasia occurs, but it can continue for weeks and even months. Fortunately, most patients recover spontaneously, especially their receptive language abilities. There are several reasons for this reaction, including gradual reduction of brain swelling, improved blood flow to deprived brain areas, adjacent areas assuming the functions of damaged ones, and a general tendency for the body to heal itself. Unfortunately, as a group, patients with **global aphasia** show little spontaneous improvement and do not benefit significantly from therapies to improve or restore their communication abilities.

Therapy for a patient with aphasia must be tailored to his or her communication strengths and weaknesses. Generally, the most intact modes of communication are used to help improve the more impaired ones. For example, if reading is a strong modality, a clinician may use it to improve the expressive recall of words by having the patient read aloud. The patient's level of motivation, family support, learning abilities, and psychological status must also be considered. Many workbooks, tapes, computer programs, flash cards, and other commercial therapeutic materials are available for aphasia therapy. In addition, there are drills and exercises for aphasia-related reading, writing, arithmetic, auditory comprehension, and verbal expression disorders.

Case Studies in Aphasia

Case Study 5.1 A 44-Year-Old Man with Traumatically Induced Jargon Aphasia and Denial-Projection

ROY

Roy's meteoric climb up the corporate ladder was legendary in the investment banking world. He was born in Detroit and spent his early years on its mean streets fending off temptation and crime. His caring parents, dedicated teachers, and an uncle who preached the power of education sparked him to achieve his potential. With the help of scholarships and student loans, Roy graduated from a prestigious business college with a master's in business administration and landed a job at one of Detroit's most aggressive international investment banks. He prided himself on giving his family the good life, as well as a strong religion and a stable home. Roy was more than a businessman; he was a family man. On weekends, he visited and cared for his elderly parents. After dinner, he met several of his buddies at the neighborhood pool hall for a few games and a couple of beers.

On this particular Saturday night the pool hall was packed with the usual neighborhood crowd drinking, boasting, laughing, and listening to loud music. Roy walked through the smoke-filled bar area to the pool tables at the rear of the room where his two longtime friends were already locked in a close game, challenged the winner, and laid his $5 bet on the edge of the pool table. He noticed two strangers admiring the custom-made cue he had brought and the cash in his wallet.

Roy was on his game that night and won nearly $500 from his friends and the two strangers. At first, Roy tempered his playing by missing a few easy shots, using a sloppy bridge, and pulling bad English. After a few beers, the games became more intense, and the betting increased. Late that night, Roy's friends left, and he and one of the strangers continued the game. Just before 2:00 a.m. the last game was played, and Roy won a hefty bet. He then unscrewed his cue, placed it carefully in its case, bid the stranger farewell, and started the short walk to his parents' home and his car.

No one knows what happened next. The police report listed him as the victim of aggravated assault, robbery, and attempted homicide. He was found lying unconscious on the sidewalk with his head bleeding profusely. The police detectives believed he had been assaulted with a blunt object, possibly the thick end of a cue stick. His wallet, minus credit cards and cash, was in a dumpster next to an adjacent bar, and his cue stick was nowhere to be found. The primary suspects, the strangers in the pool hall, were never apprehended. Several days later, in Roy's hospital room, the detectives interviewed him about the crime. They learned little about the suspects but a lot about jargon aphasia.

On Roy's chart, the diagnosis read "closed head traumatic brain injury." Radiological reports showed that the blunt blow or blows had damaged the temporal-parietal lobes of his brain. Although his head had bled, no foreign object had penetrated the brain. The computed tomography scan showed several ruptured blood vessels and damage to Wernicke's and adjacent areas of the brain. There was also bleeding (hemorrhaging) within the brain but not enough to require suctioning (evacuation). Also listed on the medical report was "jargon aphasia."

"Do you remember the assault?" asked the senior detective. Roy looked at him, smiled, and calmly replied, "It all depends on the acrylic." The detectives looked at each other quizzically. "Roy, do you know the names of the assailants?" Again Roy smiled and replied fluently: "Thusfar." Then he gestured to the table next to his bed, apparently offering the detectives a glass of water. They politely declined. "On the night of the assault, you were playing pool with friends and two strangers," stated the senior detective. "Do you know the names of the strangers?" Roy again smiled and fluently said: "It all depends on the acrylic, don't you know, and thusfar tula beyond the reef." Perplexed, the detective decided to have him describe the assailants: "How tall were the strangers?" Roy took a sip of water from the blue cup on the hospital table and laughing replied: "I'd say, thusfar, that, you know, tula is the thusfar." Then Roy chuckled. Undaunted, the first detective again asked in a much louder voice: "How tall were the strangers?" and Roy, becoming irritated, said: "Thusfar, you know!" The other detective, writing in a notebook, said: "Sir, you are not making sense." Roy looked at the senior detective and rolled his eyes, suggesting that the junior investigator was the one not making sense and needed to pay better attention.

Eventually, Roy was admitted to the hospital's rehabilitation unit. The battery of speech, language, and neuropsychological tests profiled his aphasia and related cognitive deficits, providing the basis for therapy. Often Roy refused to participate in the evaluation procedures and indicated that he was confined to the hospital for routine tests. With coaxing by his wife, Roy did participate in a token test. This test is used to assess the patient's auditory comprehension, and involve the patient matching differently colored, shaped, and sized chips based on the examiner's verbal requests. For example, the examiner might say, "Point to the red circle" and "Put the yellow square below the blue triangle." When Roy did cooperate rather than dismiss the request, he could only do the easiest task. The results of the test showed severe auditory comprehension deficits.

Clinical Sidebar 5.1
Anosognosia is ignorance, lack of awareness, or denial of disability. It usually involves paralysis but also can occur with other impairments, such as blindness and aphasia. It is associated with damage to the nondominant parietal lobe. What is the difference between denial and lack of awareness of a disease or disability?

After several weeks of poor rehabilitation gains, especially in aphasia therapy, a special examination was conducted. Roy's failure to participate in therapy was addressed and a psychiatric consultation reviewed. The psychiatrist confirmed that Roy denied his disabilities, a common reaction in patients with parietal lobe damage, and engaged in projection. According to the psychiatrist, denial is a defense mechanism used to avoid confronting negative life changes. Projection serves the same purpose and allows the patient to assign responsibility to others. Denial and projection often go hand-in-hand. The psychiatrist noted that these reactions often subside naturally, but Roy's radical psychological reactions appeared chronic. The rehabilitation team agreed that unless they could be reduced or eliminated, Roy would be discharged. According to the psychiatrist, there are no medications to eliminate denial and projection, but sometimes confrontation is helpful.

To confront Roy with his disabilities, an aphasia therapy session was videotaped. During the session, Roy was asked to name body parts, pictures of family members, and objects placed on a table. There were closeups of Roy erring, denying, projecting, and refusing to comply with the requests. After the session, the videotape was edited and reduced to about 10 minutes of relevant closeups to be used during the confrontation session.

A few days later, Roy, his wife and his oldest daughter, the psychiatrist, the speech-language pathologists, and several other members of the rehabilitation team met in the conference room to view the videotape. The atmosphere was one of support and encouragement. After the reason for the viewing was explained, the tape was played. Roy became angry and agitated, often turning away to avoid the screen. After the viewing ended, the psychiatrist asked Roy several questions about the videotape. Using convoluted jargon, Roy explained that he was not the person videotaped, and that even if he was, there was no abnormal communication whatsoever.

The attempts to jar him from denial were unsuccessful. Eventually, Roy was discharged home. Over the years his comprehension improved somewhat and the jargon speech partially diminished, but he was never able to return to his previous job and his position in his family.

Case Study 5.2   An 86-Year-Old Woman with Moderately Severe Predominantly Expressive Aphasia and Perseveration

HELEN

The residential wing of the luxurious retirement center is cozy and comfortable. The three-story building is nestled in rolling hills surrounded by acres of oak and maple trees, with manicured lawns and shorn shrubs, blending into the nearly rural suburban landscape. The affluent owners of each apartment have used their retirement savings to buy lifelong leases guaranteeing them the good life. Lush carpets, blooming flower bouquets, and expensive original paintings adorn brightly lit halls. Each floor has an oak-paneled library and a sunny solarium, and there are spas and recreational centers on the first floor. Three gourmet meals are prepared daily, and waiters serve the residents on linen tablecloths with expensive silverware. A doorman greets visitors, and there is valet parking in the underground garage. Eighty-six-year-old Helen has lived here for 9 years.

The source of Helen's vast wealth is unknown. According to some residents and staff, the seeds were sown in the crime-ridden Chicago of the 1920s, in a family business Helen ran after her husband's suspicious death. Others believe that her money is simply the result of wise investing and several bull markets. What is not debatable is that Helen is the consummate lady. She is thoughtful, polite, considerate to all, and generous to a fault. Few people know that she anonymously pays the hefty medical bills for a gardener's daughter stricken with cancer. Two months ago, she had a stroke that robbed her of language. Still, Helen has maintained her grace and dignity, and is transported to the attached rehabilitation center for daily outpatient aphasia therapy.

Helen is brought to your office by a volunteer who locks her wheelchair into place at the therapy table. Helen is dressed in a tasteful business suit, her hair is styled impeccably, and you detect a slight wisp of perfume. After sharing a few pleasantries about the weather, you get down to work. Today's session is devoted to sentence completion exercises. For Helen, the most frustrating part of aphasia is the word-finding problems, especially the perseveration. Sometimes her mind locks on a word and she cannot shake it. As usual, she earnestly attempts to complete the frustrating tasks.

You say, "Helen, please fill in the blank: 'The United States of _____.'" She smiles and clearly says, "America." You reward her with the thumbs-up gesture and the comment "Great job." Clearly pleased with herself, Helen awaits the next sentence. "Red, white, and _____." Helen again smiles and says, "America." Then, as if stung by her verbal impotence, she winces and tries to self-correct. "America, no, America, I mean . . . A . . . merica." Again she smiles and says, "Am . . . am . . . blue?" You quickly comment, "Great job; keep it up." The next sentence is provided: "Knife, fork, and _____." Helen quickly says, "America." Then in frustration she says,

Clinical Sidebar 5.2
Some perseverative-
echolalic patients benefit
from alternating serial
drills that require shifting
from one word to the
next. For example, the
clinician names the first
day (Monday) in the
days of the week. The
patient then names the
next day (Tuesday), the
clinician the third day
(Wednesday), and so
forth. The goal is for the
patient with echolalia to
resist the tendency to
say the last word heard.
The therapy can also
involve other series of
words such as the
months of the year,
counting, and spelling.
What is the difference
between perseveration
and echolalia?

"No, no, no!" The majority of the session is filled with the frustration of naming errors compounded by perseveration.

Knowing that these frustrating exercises can cause anxiety and possibly a panic attack, several times during the session you stop the exercises and engage in chitchat. Verbal impotence can be very threatening to a patient's self-esteem. To lessen the stress, you show pictures and have Helen discuss them with no pressure to produce correct responses. One picture shows dancers apparently doing the Charleston, the rage of the 1920s and 1930s. Helen points to the picture and says, "Flapper."

Aware that neurogenic communication disorders can evolve into different types, at first you suspect that she has uttered a made-up word, a neologism. Perhaps *flap* approximates *tap,* as in *tap dance,* and *er,* as in *dancer.* But Helen's response is inconsistent with her predominantly expressive aphasia because she had not displayed any form of jargon in the past. Again Helen says, "Flapper" and, even more curiously, points to herself, apparently proud of the statement. During the remaining sentence completion exercises, Helen continues to improve in naming and overcoming the perseveration. Several times, however, *flapper* is perseverately inserted into the drills.

With some free time before the next session, you decide to search the World Wide Web for *flapper* in an attempt to understand Helen's curious symptoms. Perhaps you are simply not aware of the meaning of the term. To your surprise, there are several references to the word and descriptions of wild women who danced the Charleston with clothing and jewelry flapping. During the roaring 20s and 30s, flappers danced at speakeasies where illegal beer flowed and good times were had during the Prohibition era. Chicago's gangster-run South Side was home to many speakeasies, flappers, and profitable rum-running businesses. Apparently, fortunes were made during prohibition, and you recall the rumors of Helen's vast wealth and ponder this interesting woman's past.

Case Study 5.3 A 46-Year-Old Woman with Predominantly Expressive Aphasia and Telegraphic Speech as a Complication of Heart Surgery

CHARLENE

The restaurant is the hub of the small town and surrounding farms. It is where townspeople discuss political issues during early morning breakfasts, lunch with each other at midday, and feast on large T-bone and ribeye steaks in the evening. The bar next to the dining room is the favorite watering hole on weekends. With her sister's help, Charlene has run the prosperous establishment for nearly 10 years. Twelve-hour days of planning meals and deliveries, supervising cooks and servers, and paying bills are the norm, and Charlene never complains. At 46, she seems to have endless energy and a commitment to the thriving business. Lately, though, she has felt more tired than usual, and dizziness brought her to the hospital one evening. Over the next week, several tests confirm a heart valve irregularity and the need for surgery.

Charlene knows that the best medical services are usually found at teaching hospitals. These hospitals usually conduct more research, have greater financial resources and better-trained staff, and more experience with a particular medical specialty. Because of the delicate heart surgery Charlene needs, her family wants the best. This involves traveling to the city, arranging temporary accommodations, and closing the restaurant for nearly a month. Charlene is understandably nervous, especially when she signs the paperwork acknowledging the risks involved in the surgery, including stroke and death, and releasing the doctors and hospital from liability. At surgery, the doctors, nurses, technicians, and anesthesiologist do a commendable job. Charlene returns home, reopens the restaurant, and continues her life, albeit at a slower pace. It seems that the ordeal is over.

Clinical Sidebar 5.3
Sentence expansion exercises help some patients with telegraphic speech to create longer, grammatically correct utterances. When the patient produces telegraphic speech, the clinician uses a hand gesture as a cue to "stretch out" the utterance. For example, if the patient says, "Eat now," the clinician uses the gesture. The patient then says, "I want to eat now," followed by verbal praise from the clinician. For some patients, the clinician may have to model the desired utterance. Do you believe telegraphic speech is a grammatical disorder or the result of an impoverished vocabulary?

One Sunday morning, as Charlene gets up from her lawn chair to refill her cup of coffee, her right hand fails to grasp the cup. It crashes to the patio floor and she utters something unintelligible to her sister. An ambulance rushes her to the nearest hospital, tests are run, and the diagnosis is confirmed. Charlene has had a stroke.

The doctor explains to her sister that a clot has obstructed blood flow to parts of the left hemisphere of Charlene's brain. The clot probably originated in the heart and traveled to the brain. The doctor believes that the heart surgery caused the clot, either directly or indirectly. He notes the occasional premature contraction or "flutter" in her heartbeat, a condition that sometimes causes clots to form, despite the medications used to prevent them. Charlene has Broca's aphasia and will need extensive rehabilitation.

Charlene's aphasia primarily involves expressive language. At first, she did not understand some of the words spoken by others, especially when people spoke rapidly or used complex words. However, over a 2-week period, this problem subsided. Expressively, Charlene uses primarily telegraphic speech, in which the minimum number of function words, such as conjunctions, adjectives, and articles, and many content words, such as nouns and verbs, are used to express an idea. This condition is likely the result of her general impoverishment of words.

Charlene's telegraphic speech is part of a larger class of language disorders called *agrammatism* or *syntactic aphasia*, in which the patient has problems producing words in their correct sequence and with proper grammar. Besides telegraphic speech,

Charlene had difficultly with prepositions. The stroke appears to have eliminated her ability to understand and use correctly words such as *over, under, above, below,* and so forth. However, her telegraphic speech is the primary manifestation of the predominantly expressive aphasia.

On the first day of aphasia therapy, the clinician asks Charlene to describe the events surrounding her stroke. Using telegraphic speech, she says, "My sister, uh, coffee the patio. Ducks . . . creek. Crash coffee floor. Oh my God! What's wrong. Talk to me. Talk to me. No can talk. Go hospital. Talk to me! My sister, uh. Charlene, talk to me! Here I be."

During the weeks of therapy, Charlene's expressive vocabulary improves, especially for function words and prepositions, and the telegraphic utterances are nearly eliminated. Even when she uses telegraphic speech, it is more complex and includes more function words. Eventually, Charlene is able to return to her home and resume management of the restaurant.

Case Study 5.4 A 68-Year-Old Man with Predominantly Receptive Aphasia and Auditory-Acoustic Agnosia

BLAIR

Blair preferred to be called a *character actor.* He has a long list of credits to his name and has played hundreds of supporting roles in plays, in movies, and on television. Long ago he accepted the fact that people would say, "Aren't you in the movies?" while never remembering his name. Blair has never been plagued by hordes of fans seeking an autograph. He started to act at age 7, when his parents moved to California to work in the technical trades of the burgeoning movie industry. He first worked as an extra and then took bit parts with three or four lines. As he grew older, the jobs became more plentiful and his agent, a crusty ex-stuntman with great movie business sense, keep him in nearly full-time employment. During his 30s and 40s, Blair took several supporting roles as a cowboy; many of these movies were shot in the beautiful towering red rocks of Sedona, Arizona. Later in life, along with many other actors, artists, and celebrities, he returned to Sedona to retire.

Celia and Blair married when they were in their early 20s. Throughout their marriage, Celia was the sensible business manager, a role Blair gladly avoided. She negotiated and purchased their California and Arizona homes, invested wisely, and focused on the practical side of life. Blair was the consummate artist, creative and often oblivious to practical realities. One of their friends said Celia was the logical left hemisphere and Blair the creative right hemisphere to their brain union. Celia was a self-taught businessperson, and when Blair suffered his stroke, she decided to educate herself. She listened intently to the doctors and specialists as they described Blair's brain damage and symptoms, searched the Internet, and spent hours in libraries searching medical books and journals for information about strokes and their devastating effect on the ability to communicate. When she called the speech and

thought, and his question catches you off-guard. You promise to research it and let him know.

Once the skin has been parted and cauterized to stop the bleeding, four holes are drilled into the skull. The drill is a sophisticated neurosurgical instrument costing thousands of dollars, but the shinny drill bit, trigger, and lugging, whirring sound remind you of your portable Black and Decker. The drill holes, about one third of an inch in diameter, form the corner borders of a square. Another sophisticated neurosurgical device, reminding you of your Black and Decker portable reciprocating saw, is carefully inserted into one of the holes and, as in a game of connect-the-dots, the skull is carefully straight-cut from hole to hole. The sawed section is about the size of a computer mouse. The neurosurgeon carefully removes the cut section of skull and places it in a tray of liquid. Because of the pressure caused by the tumor, the surface of Lou's brain bulges out from the hole.

That evening, you go to the library to find the answer. You search the literature for aphasia and negatives, affirmatives, closed-end questions, anomia, dysnomia, confrontation naming errors, word retrieval, and so forth. After analyzing the studies and articles, you finally discover the likely answer.

The membranes covering the brain are carefully and precisely cut and retracted. Then the surgeon begins spreading brain tissue and peeling back gray matter until the cancerous mass is revealed. A long, narrow probe is inserted, and the tumorous mass is excised and evacuated. A loud suctioning sound is heard as the surgeon carefully moves the probe from one area to another. The probe vibrates at an ultrasonic frequency that dislodges the mass but spares the healthy, more resilient and inviolable tissue. Soon most (hopefully, all) of the out-of-control cells have been removed and the process of closing begins. The three membranes are replaced, and the square skull bone is sutured into position. Finally, Lou's skin is sewn back into place, and the anesthesiologist brings him back to consciousness. The operation is deemed a success, and the patient is taken to the recovery room.

Lou awaits the answer to his question. You explain that aphasic word-finding errors often involve verbal paraphasias—unintended substitution of one word for another from the same category of words. In this condition, the unintended word is associated semantically with the desired, correct one. Yes and no are associated, one-word, closed-end responses to questions. You explain to Lou that when he inadvertently and incorrectly says "No" for "Yes" and vice versa, the mistake is this type of error. Lou accepts the answer and appears relieved that you know he is not chronically ambivalent. You and Lou continue with exercises to improve the accuracy of yes and no, but now with the knowledge that this is simply an example of the types of naming errors that typically occur in aphasia.

Clinical Sidebar 5.5
Several diseases and disorders cause progressive deterioration of speech and language. There is little spontaneous recovery, and the disorder becomes increasingly severe. Nevertheless, therapies and treatments are justified if the rate of deterioration is slowed and short-term gains can be demonstrated. How might progressive disorders create special problems for the grieving patient in accepting the situation?

Case Study 5.6   A 69-Year-Old Man with Global Aphasia

LEROY

Your diagnosis in the nursing home chart reads: "Global aphasia and right hemi-paralysis secondary to a cerebrovascular accident." The radiology reports show that both Broca's and Wernicke's areas have been severely damaged by an obstruction to the left middle cerebral artery. You are confined to a wheelchair, but by carefully moving your left foot and arm, you can move fairly directly. Sometimes you use your left hand to grasp the rail along the corridors to go from one place to another. Over the past 4 years, you have become a familiar figure in the halls, lounges, and dining rooms of this large medical care facility.

The massive stroke has destroyed most of your speech and language. The only purposeful verbal expressions you are capable of uttering are "Uh" and "Kayla," and these are used interchangeably for a variety of requests. Words spoken by others sound like a strange foreign language. You can no longer read or write. However, you are still capable of understanding basic gestures such as a handshake, and you can turn away to show avoidance and refusal. The entire right side of your body is paralyzed, including your face.

At first, you were devastated by the stroke and aphasia. You have always been fit, strong, and active. The only other time you were hospitalized was when you were born, and now you live your final days in this institution, removed from your home and your wife of 45 years. Even when your family visits, the bridge of communication has collapsed and the aphasia prevents discussions of the life you once shared. The stroke and global aphasia have separated you psychologically and physically from your loved ones. It took many months of grieving, but you now accept life's new realities. You have adjusted to the unwanted changes.

In this nursing home, life revolves around the three meals. You are awakened at 7:00 a.m. for breakfast. Because you have a history of depression, the staff prefers that you eat in the dining room. They want you to dress and socialize with the other patients rather than eat alone in your room. Because of the paralysis, you need help to dress, but thanks to occupational therapy, you can comb your hair, brush your teeth, and take care of basic bathroom activities. Although the kind nurses' aides always offer to push you in your wheelchair to the dining room, you insist on doing it yourself. When they offer, you refuse by politely saying, "Kayla" and "Uh, Kayla" and begin the time-consuming task of independent movement. After breakfast, some of the residents do activities or therapies, but most end up in the television area next to the nurses' station.

During lunch, the dining room is packed with patients and staff. Usually, the staff sit with each other and their jobs can be clearly discerned by the color of their uniforms. The patients dine with each other, and many require assistance cutting their food and moving it to their lips; some need help and monitoring when they swallow. Although nursing home food is usually notoriously bad, here, the meals are healthy and surprisingly tasty. And thanks to occupational therapy, you can use utensils with large, fat handles and can feed yourself chopped and soft meals. After lunch, most residents return to their rooms or the television area or simply wander the halls. You usually return to the empty dining room and sit at a table at the rear. You enjoy watching the kitchen staff coming and going, the weather changes through the large windows, and private time for yourself. Privacy is hard to find in a nursing home. It was during one of these solitary times that you rescued a woman from certain frostbite and received acclaim for doing it. You are the home's hero for a day.

It is mid-February, and the snow has been falling for several days. The snowdrifts are high and the wind is howling. You watch the snow swirl around the walls of the building. The warmth of the dining room is in stark contrast to the arctic outdoors, giving you a pleasant sense of security and comfort.

Nineteen-year-old Margaret Hunter is in her second week of employment at the nursing home. She took the job as a dishwasher to pay her share of the rent in the new apartment she and her two high school friends have just rented. Money is tight, and to help make ends meet, she has also decided to quit smoking. However, she never realized how difficult it would be. One of her jobs in the kitchen is to scrub surfaces until they are clean. As she works, she feels the intense nicotine urge. She has cut down to five or six cigarettes a day and thinks that now is the time for her afternoon fix. Smoking is prohibited in the facility, so she must stand outside with other smoking outcasts or use her car on inclement days. Today, however, time is short, and she decides to stand just outside the large door and smoke briefly to calm her nerves. She walks past one of the familiar patients and waves to him. His name is LeRoy, and he seems pleasant and friendly. She suspects that he has had a stroke and knows that he cannot talk. As she opens the large self-locking glass door, a blast of cold air enters the room. She stands just outside with her foot holding it open a crack, lights the cigarette, and puffs away. Then she slips on the ice, and the door closes behind her. The only other entrance is at the front of the massive building, past several fences and through the parking lot. She shakes the door and knocks several times on the window. The only person in the dining room is LeRoy, and she wonders if he has the ability to help. After all, he has brain damage and even drools. Margaret stands outside in the freezing cold with only her uniform to protect her.

Clinical Sidebar 5.6
The public and even some professionals sometimes believe that patients with global aphasia are severely cognitively impaired. They treat them as if they are children, retarded, or demented. Patients with global aphasia are not reduced to childlike states, nor do they have dementia or mental retardation, even though they may only be able to communicate with a few words or gestures. How is inner speech related to intelligence?

You watch Margaret leave the dining room, open the door, light the cigarette, and begin smoking. Although you have no inner speech to verbally structure your thoughts, you understand and appreciate her situation. You too smoked for many years. You suspect that she must be cold and getting colder when you see and hear the door slam closed. She begins knocking on the door and beckons to you to open it.

Although your massive stroke has destroyed your speaking, reading, writing, and verbal understanding, it has not rendered you mentally retarded or senile. You still process information visually, and can appreciate circumstances and solve problems.

Your memories of life experiences are largely intact, and your kind, caring personality still exists. Although the stroke and aphasia have destroyed your ability to abstract verbally, verbal abstraction is not necessary to appreciate a cold woman's desperate need, maneuver the wheelchair to the door, firmly press down on the bar with your left hand, weather a blast of cold air, and accept a chilly hug from a grateful smoker.

Case Study 5.7   A 55-Year-Old Woman with Aphasia and Severe Depression

RUTH

The rehabilitation team meetings are held in the third-floor conference room. The meeting is held every Tuesday, starting promptly at 7:30 a.m. Agendas have been provided, and the physiatrist sits at the head of the conference table. Soon professionals from many disciplines take their usual places at the table, and the meeting begins. Ruth is the first patient on the agenda.

The physiatrist summarizes Ruth's current medical status. She is a white 55-year-old clinical psychologist with a history of diabetes. Several members of the team saw her while she was in the acute care wing of the hospital, and she has been in the rehabilitation unit for 14 days. The patient suffered a dense thrombotic cerebrovascular accident as a result of occlusion to the left middle cerebral artery. The radiology report shows brain damage to Broca's area in the posterior inferior left frontal lobe and surrounding areas, including the insula. Ruth has right hemiparalysis and aphasia and was incontinent for a while.

The physical therapist reviews Ruth's progress in learning to transfer from wheelchair to bed and to use a walker. The patient is having little success. Two days ago, she fell in the physical therapy gym but was not seriously hurt, and an incident report was filed. The therapist notes that the range of motion of Ruth's arm is severely reduced, and its occasional spastic contractions are painful. He also says that Ruth is lethargic and often is only partially motivated. Using the hospital's rehabilitation rating system, he says that Ruth continues to function at a 2.5 level. Unfortunately, he believes that the goal of 4.0, semi-independent movement and transfers, will not be met.

The occupational therapist also suggests that Ruth is less than enthusiastic about relearning the activities of daily living. This therapist has substituted Velcro for zippers and shoelaces, but Ruth continues to have difficulty dressing herself. Independent eating is also problematic. Although some movement is returning to Ruth's right hand, she is very clumsy in using it. She prefers to use her left hand during meals but is quite awkward. The therapist gives Ruth a 2.0 and also questions whether she will meet the initial occupational therapy rehabilitation goals.

The social worker reports that Ruth's financial situation is adequate. She has good insurance coverage, but the out-of-pocket expenses will be considerable. Apparently she will be able to pay them. Ruth has one daughter living in a distant state. Initially, a few friends visited occasionally, but the patient has little consistent social and emotional support. The social worker says that Ruth is lethargic and aloof.

The speech-language pathologist notes that Ruth's receptive abilities have improved considerably since her first visit in the intensive care unit. The clinician reviews the results of the recently administered token test, in which the patient followed commands by pointing to or rearranging differently colored and shaped objects. The results show that Ruth can understand the speech of others. "Expressively, Ruth has some problems sequencing and planning muscle movement to produce speech, but retrieving the words from memory is the main aspect of the disorder," the therapist reports. Both finding the correct word and then planning and programming it are problematic. Using professional jargon, she says, "The patient has Broca's aphasia with a preponderance of anomia." Ruth is given the same numerical rating she received last week, showing little if any improvement. However, the clinician notes Ruth's improved right-hand motor functioning and reports that this is accompanied by increased expressive communication in many patients.

Then the clinician asks the physiatrist if she would consider prescribing an antidepressant. Ruth is extremely depressed, and the condition is not resolving. The clinician explains that the antidepressant will help increase Ruth's motivation and her ability to benefit from therapy. The clinician knows that depression and anxiety are common in patients with this type of aphasia, possibly caused by changes in brain chemistry resulting from the stroke. The stress and loss associated with the disabilities also contribute to the depression. The fact that Ruth lacks consistent emotional and social support from family and friends is also persuasive. The neuropsychologist concurs and says, "It's hard to learn to navigate in a storm. Antidepressants calm the seas long enough for the patient to mobilize adaptive defenses and workable coping mechanisms." The physiatrist agrees and notes that if the depression is primarily organic, that is, caused by the brain damage, the antidepressant regimen may be of long duration, perhaps permanent. It depends on whether the brain's chemistry can be readjusted. She also notes that antidepressants should never be a quick and easy fix for the complex disturbances caused by stroke and aphasia, but they have a place in rehabilitation and are remarkably free of serious side effects.

Clinical Sidebar 5.7
Many studies have shown the value of aphasia therapy. With the possible exception of those with global aphasia, most patients with aphasia benefit from speech and language therapy. They improve more rapidly, in broader dimensions, and ultimately recover more of their communication abilities than those who do not receive therapy. Patients and their families report that one of the greatest benefits of therapy is in the psychological domain. Therapy helps patients deal with the many unwanted changes caused by the aphasia and cope with the disorder. Can therapy be justified if the patient can learn only four or five words?

SUMMARY

Aphasia is the loss of previously acquired language abilities due to a neurological insult; to varying degrees, it affects all modalities of communication. Two forms of aphasia can occur: predominantly expressive and predominantly receptive. Mild aphasia may only be a nuisance, producing occasional word-finding problems and difficulty understanding long, complex statements. Global aphasia can render a patient mute and unable to read, write, gesture, and understand the speech of others. Some patients with aphasia may experience organic depression, anxiety, perseveration, emotional lability, and the grief response. Most patients with aphasia benefit from therapy, relearn speech and language, or learn alternative ways to communicate.

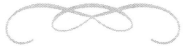

Study and Discussion Questions

1. List and describe the symptoms of expressive and receptive aphasia. Discuss how each modality of communication can be impaired.

2. Compare and contrast aphasia resulting from stroke and traumatic brain injury.

3. Compare and contrast aphasia and agnosia.

4. What is a catastrophic reaction, and how might a clinician accidentally cause it?

5. Describe the symptoms of aphasia. How does awareness of the disability affect the prognosis?

6. How do organic and grieving depression differ in aphasia?

7. Provide five examples of telegraphic speech and the longer sentences from which they are derived.

8. How can providing incorrect "yes/no" answers be considered verbal paraphasia?

9. Compare and contrast the cognitive abilities of patients with global aphasia and those of individuals with profound mental impairment–mental retardation.

10. List the typical members of a rehabilitation team and discuss their responsibilities.

Recommended Reading

Darley, F. (1982). *Aphasia*. Philadelphia: Saunders.

This classic textbook provides a comprehensive overview of aphasia. It clearly separates neurogenic language impairments from nonlanguage motor speech disorders.

Davis, G. A. (2000). *Aphasiology: Disorders and clinical practice*. Boston: Allyn & Bacon.

This book provides a summary of aphasia and an overview of specific symptoms.

Huttlinger, K., & Tanner, D. (1994). The peyote way: Implications for culture care nursing. *Journal of Transcultural Nursing, 5*(2), 5–11.

This article provides a case study of aphasia and a peyote healing ceremony.

Tanner, D. (1999). *The family guide to surviving stroke and communication disorders.* Austin: PRO-ED.

This book addresses the nature of aphasia and related disorders and includes "The Aphasic Patient's Bill of Rights."

Tanner, D. (2003). *Exploring communication disorders: A 21st century introduction through literature and media.* Boston: Allyn & Bacon.

Read Chapter 8 for a review of aphasia using references to public figures, movies, television shows, and a Broadway play.

Tanner, D. (2003). *The psychology of neurogenic communication disorders: A primer for health care professionals.* Boston: Allyn & Bacon.

This book discusses neurogenic communication disorders and explores coping styles and defense mechanisms. Read the short story "Murphy's Inner World of Aphasia" for a first-person account of aphasia and its effects on a patient and his family.

CHAPTER SIX

Motor Speech Disorders

Disease often tells its secrets in a casual parenthesis.

Wilfred Trotter

Chapter Preview: In this chapter, the motor speech disorders of apraxia of speech and the dysarthrias are examined. There is a review of motor speech programming and the five basic motor speech processes. Respiration, phonation-resonance, articulation, and prosody are discussed, emphasizing the effects certain diseases and disorders have on them. The case studies include communication disorders associated with apraxia of speech and several dysarthrias. There is also a case study of alleged medical malpractice involving a child born with spastic cerebral palsy.

OVERVIEW OF MOTOR SPEECH PRODUCTION AND DISORDERS

In *motor speech disorders, motor* refers to the neural structures causing muscle fibers to contract. These disorders include pathologies of the motor cortex, the nerves (efferent, descending nerve fibers), and the muscles involved in speech production. Clinicians also refer to these types of disorders as **neuromuscular** speech disorders. Hundreds, if not thousands, of neurological deficits and diseases can cause motor speech disorders. Before the mid-1970s, college courses on motor speech disorders addressed particular diseases or defects such as cerebral palsy, multiple sclerosis, or muscular dystrophy; alternatively, several of these conditions were covered in an umbrella course on organic disorders. In 1975, Darley, Aronson, and Brown at the Mayo Clinic in Rochester, Minnesota, provided a classification system based on the level of neuromuscular impairments in their landmark book *Motor Speech Disorders.* Today, motor speech disorders are divided into apraxia of speech and six types of dysarthrias based on their classification system. This system has not changed significantly except for Duffy's (1995) addition of **unilateral upper motor neuron dysarthria.** ח (ש

Darley and colleagues' classification system of neurogenic communication disorders has been widely accepted by clinicians from a variety of disciplines. Besides providing a logical and efficient way of classifying motor speech disorders, it dramatically influenced aphasiology. Although in the past some authorities had proposed detailed classification systems for neurogenic communication disorders, clinicians typically included them in adult language disorders. The boundaries between language and motor speech disorders were blurred, leading to unfortunate labels such as *motor aphasia* and *sensorimotor aphasia*. Perhaps the biggest problem caused by including motor speech disorders in aphasia classification systems involved clinical practice. Although the symptoms, objectives, and methods overlap, aphasia is a language disorder distinctly different from the motor speech disorders and requires different therapies.

Symbolic and Nonsymbolic Neurogenic Communication Disorders

When addressing neurogenic communication disorders, it is convenient to separate them into **symbolic** and **nonsymbolic** impairments. Symbolic disorders impair or eliminate verbal symbolic processing. A symbol is an **arbitrary** representation of reality, and the word, whether spoken, gestured, or written, is a linguistic symbol. Certain neurological diseases and disorders can impair or destroy verbal symbolic processing. Neurogenic communication disorders that impair or destroy language are aphasia, the language of confusion resulting from traumatic brain injury, psychotic language, and the generalized intellectual impairments seen in dementia.

Nonsymbolic neurogenic communication disorders are **apraxia of speech** and the **dysarthrias**. Although these disorders can co-occur with symbolic disorders, in their pure form they do not disrupt or impair symbolism. In addition, motor disorders are influenced by **sensory** impairments that also may result from neurological deficits and diseases. Apraxia of speech is the inability to perform voluntary movements not resulting from impaired comprehension or paralysis. Technically, patients with **dyspraxia** maintain some ability to speak. Clinicians use the term *apraxia of speech* to refer to both the total inability and the impaired ability to produce voluntary speech. At the highest level of motor speech programming, the symbol (word meaning) **intersects** with the articulatory program; each word contains the program for its utterance.

Motor Speech Programming and Apraxia of Speech

There are three levels of neurological impairment and resulting apraxias of speech. At the conceptual level, **ideational apraxia** of speech results from the speaker's inability to grasp the thought driving the speech act. This type of apraxia of speech is seen in dementia and other cognitive-linguistic disorders in which the patient has trouble conceptualizing the idea driving an utterance. (In ideational apraxia of speech, there is no clear discrimination between symbolic and nonsymbolic processing.) At the speech planning level, the utterance's motor plan is formulated, including articulatory timing, speed, and strength. This type of apraxia, sometimes called **ideomotor apraxia**, most closely resembles the apraxia of speech described by Darely et al. discussed below. At the planning level the motor speech (articulatory) program is created, and at the activation level the plan is set in motion. During activation, the neural commands are sent to the muscles of the speech mechanism and the neuromotor requirements for the utterance are met. In this type of apraxia, sometimes called **motor apraxia**, execution of the movement is defective. Table 6.1 shows the three levels of motor speech programming and apraxias of speech.

Table 6.1 Levels of Neurological Impairments and Apraxia of Speech

Neurological Level	Apraxia of Speech	Manifestations
Conceptual	Ideational	Difficulty integrating the speech act into the concept
Formulation	Ideomotor	Difficulty formulating and programming the motor plan for voluntary speech acts
Execution	Motor	Impaired performance, integration, and sequencing of voluntary speech movements

Clinical Patterns of Apraxia of Speech

Patients with apraxia of speech **complicate** the speech act. In this sense, apraxia of speech resembles the effortful compensatory behaviors of stuttering. One feature of apraxia of speech is the dichotomy between voluntary and involuntary speech. When utterances are automatic and overlearned, they can sometimes be said easily and normally. By contrast, propositional, voluntary, thoughtful, and purposeful utterances result in **verbal impotence**. Speech programmed and executed with little forethought is called *automatic speech.*

Because repeated speech is propositional, voluntary, thoughtful, and purposeful, impaired repetition is often a hallmark of apraxia of speech and can be a diagnostic feature of the disorder (Tanner & Culbertson, 1999b). Patients also tend to **perseverate** on apraxic utterances and while struggling to create the proper programming. They may also insert the **schwa vowel**, another similarity between stuttering and apraxia of speech. Because apraxia of speech is a nonsymbolic neurogenic communication disorder, patients are aware of their errors but are often unable to self-correct, particularly when the disorder is severe. Programming the initial aspects of an utterance usually involves more error than subsequent aspects of the speech act.

Treatment of Apraxia of Speech

In aphasia, the goals of therapy are to relearn and deblock language. Aspects of expressive and receptive grammar, syntax, phonology, and semantics are targeted for treatment. While motor speech programming deficits are frequently a part of expressive aphasia, the treatment of apraxia of speech involves motor speech, not language. As a practical clinical matter, the goals, objectives, and treatment methods for aphasia and apraxia of speech may overlap; however, voluntary motor speech, control is the goal of apraxia of speech therapy. Treating apraxia of speech in patients who also have significant aphasia is challenging. Patients with aphasia have difficulty comprehending instructions and have expressive language deficits, creating communication barriers that interfere with learning. Concomitant disorders such as perseveration, echolalia, and emotional lability also interfere with apraxia of speech therapies.

Duffy (1995) considers **drill** an important aspect of apraxia of speech treatment: "Virtually every specific behavioral treatment approach for AOS [apraxia of speech]

emphasizes drill" (p. 421). Apraxia of speech therapy assumes that the patient has lost memory for planning, sequencing, and executing motor speech acts. Repeatedly performing these acts helps the patient to recall and relearn them. The motor acts should begin with simple speech acts and gradually increase to more complex ones. Repetition is also fundamental in treating apraxia of speech using **melodic intonation therapy** (Sparks, Helm, & Albert, 1974). In this therapy, a rhythm or melody is applied to an utterance, causing it to be programmed, sequenced, and executed more easily; then the melody is gradually reduced and eventually eliminated. (This is another similarity between apraxia of speech and stuttering.) Other therapies for apraxia of speech include the initial use of whispering, sentence completion exercises, shifting from automatic to purposeful utterances, and using nonverbal gestures to facilitate purposeful utterances. Conventional therapies for patients with nonfluent aphasia can also be applied to apraxia of speech. No therapies for apraxia of speech have been shown to help all patients, and careful ongoing assessment is needed to decide if a particular patient is benefitting from treatment.

Dysarthria and the Motor Speech Processes

In severe apraxia of speech, the patient may be unable to program respiration, phonation, and articulation for purposeful speech. Apraxia of speech is usually limited to problems with programming the articulators; the other aspects of motor speech are unimpaired or minimally disrupted. However, the dysarthrias generally disrupt one or more of the five basic motor speech processes: **respiration**, **phonation**, **articulation**, **resonance**, and **prosody** (Darley et al., 1975). Respiration provides the support for speech production. Phonation and resonance are the sound source and resonating system, respectively, of the speech production mechanism. Articulation involves shaping the oral tract to create recognizable speech sounds, and prosody is the stress, intonation, rhythm, and fluency of speech that extend across one or more segments of an utterance.

Dysarthria and Respiratory Support

Respiration, as noted above, serves as a **driving force** for speech production. Compressed air from the lungs displaces anatomical structures, and the air is forced through constrictions to produce speech sounds. The respiratory system works similarly to a **bellow**; the size of the thorax is changed to vary the pressure in the lungs. Inhalation is the rush of air from regions of high pressure to regions of low pressure; exhalation is the opposite. Respiration operates on **Boyle's law** and the **kinetic theory of gases** (Zemlin, 1998), describing air movement from regions of differing pressure.

Severe generalized dysarthrias affect the respiratory system, disrupting the driving force for speech. **Mixed** and **multiple dysarthrias**, such as those occurring in amyotrophic lateral sclerosis, multiple sclerosis, and other progressive neurological diseases, ultimately impair the muscles of respiration so that patients can no longer expand and contract the thorax adequately for speech. When respiratory support for speech production is impaired, patients tend to speak at a slow rate, with short phrasing, and with prolonged intervals between syllables, words, and phrases. In addition, during normal speech, the respiratory system adjusts for impedance variations in the oral tract. With greater impedance to airflow, such as occurs with obstruent consonants, the respiratory system must adjust for the increased resistance by reducing the force of muscular contractions. Without this adjustment, speech is produced with excess and inappropriate stress.

In some patients with severely compromised respiration, **velopharyngeal incompetence** exacerbates the lack of respiratory support. Because the patient cannot effectively seal off the nasal cavity, air leaks from the oral cavity. In feeble and weak patients, this air leakage reduces the pressure behind articulatory valves, decreasing **intelligibility**.

Patients with severely compromised respiration often have **tracheotomies** and are maintained on **respirators** or **ventilators**. Speech is possible with some types of **tracheotomies**, and some patients can "mouth" words. An electrolarynx can also provide a sound source. Writing and gestures are other avenues of communication. Therapy for patients with reduced breath support includes postural changes, the use of clavicular breathing, and exercises to maximize inhalation and control exhalation. Air wastage is also a problem when patients release air before initiating phonation. Therapy to maximize the use of breath support is necessary for these patients. In some patients, a Velcro waistband (girdle) can be used around the abdomen to maximize breath support during speech. The waistband should be removed periodically to allow the necessary deep breathing.

Phonation-Resonance Pathologies

As discussed in Chapter 4, the speech mechanism can be viewed as a sound-source resonator. The vocal cords are the sound source, and the neck and head are the resonating chambers. The frequency and amplitude of vocal cord vibrations interact with the resonance characteristics of the neck and head resonating chambers, creating acoustic energy that radiates out during speech. Some bands of energy from the sound source are amplified, whereas others are damped. Alterations in the size, shape, and length of the oral-nasal cavity create speech sounds by changing the acoustic properties of the energy coming from the glottis. (Unvoiced sounds are also a result of acoustic changes produced by the alterations of the sound source in the resonating chamber.) Although phonation and resonance are interdependent systems, it is clinically important to examine the dysarthrias resulting from laryngeal paralysis and velopharyngeal incompetence separately.

Laryngeal Paralysis

Laryngeal paralysis frequently occurs in **spastic** and **flaccid dysarthrias** due to upper and lower motor neuron impairments. Spastic laryngeal paralysis is due to bilateral upper motor neuron damage. Clinically, spasticity likely results in a harsh voice quality due to the hyperadduction of the vocal cords. However, Darley et al. (1975) found **breathiness** to be a voice characteristic in many of these patients. Duffy (1995) proposes that the breathiness is a result of **compensation**: "This breathiness could reflect a degree of vocal cord weakness, but could also represent a compensatory response rather than a primary problem" (p. 136). In some patients, breathiness rather than harshness results from attempts to avoid laryngeal constriction. When upper motor neuron damage affects phonation, it usually causes harshness and, infrequently, decreased loudness. The neurological bases for these impairments are unknown (Duffy, 1995).

Flaccid dysphonia is found in lower motor neuron damage, particularly when the **vagus nerve** (cranial nerve X) is damaged. The paralysis may involve adduction or abduction and may be bilateral or unilateral. When one or both of the vocal cords are paralyzed, they are usually fixed in the **paramedian position**, that is, near the midline of the glottis. However, this fixation does not always occur; in some patients, it is found in a more abducted position. The relative abduction or adduction fixation largely accounts for the perceptual feature of the voice. The more abducted the vocal cords, the more likely the perceptual feature is to be **breathy**; the more adducted the vocal cords, the more likely the feature is to be **harsh** and **strained**. In unilateral adductor paralysis, the perceptual features depend on the ability of the unaffected vocal cord to cross the glottal midline and contact the affected vocal cord. This principle is the basis for voice therapy in which straining and forcing exercises cause the unaffected vocal cord to cross the midline.

Cerebellar and extrapyramidal nervous system damage can also affect the laryngeal valve. Cerebellar damage causes **ataxic** (coordination) phonatory disturbances, and extrapyramidal damage results in **kinetic** (motion or movement) disorders. Although a harsh voice quality may result from cerebellar and extrapyramidal damage, pitch and loudness instability are often the most prominent phonatory deficits. Impaired respiratory-phonatory synergy likely causes ataxic phonatory disturbances (Zwirner, Murry, & Woodson, 1991). Rapid and slow unwanted phonatory movements, as well as the voice tremor seen in Parkinson's disease, are the most common perceptual features of extrapyramidal disorders (Tosi, Tanner, & Supal, 1976). Laryngeal coordination and movement therapies for laryngeal disorders are provided during dynamic speech focusing on the timing, speed, and integration of phonatory muscle movements.

Velopharyngeal Incompetence

Neuromuscular dysfunctions involving the velopharyngeal port result in phonation-resonance disorders. To varying degrees, all of the dysarthrias—flaccid, spastic, ataxic, hyperkinetic, and hypokinetic—can prevent the velum from approximating the posterior pharyngeal wall during speech. **Velopharyngeal incompetence** in dysarthria results in **hypernasality**, **audible nasal emission**, and **reduced intraoral air pressure**. Hypernasality, the excessive nasal resonance on nonnasal sounds, occurs because the velum does not approximate the posterior pharyngeal wall. Hypernasality also occurs during connected speech (**assimilated hypernasality**) because slow, sluggish velopharyngeal closure allows nasal contamination of nonnasal sounds. In assimilated hypernasality, since the velopharyngeal port does not close in a timely manner, nonnasal sounds are produced with nasalization. Audible nasal emission is the escape of air through the nasal port during the production of pressure phonemes. As discussed above, velopharyngeal incompetence causes reduced intraoral air pressure on the production of obstruent phonemes. It can reduce speech intelligibility, especially in weak patients.

In many patients with progressive neuromuscular disorders such as Parkinson's disease, amyotrophic lateral sclerosis, and multiple sclerosis, reduction of hypernasality as a speech perceptual feature is secondary to increasing intraoral air pressure to improve speech intelligibility. Several appliances are available to force the velum to continually approximate the posterior pharyngeal wall. Although continual closure of the velopharyngeal port results in denasality, it often raises the intraoral air pressure necessary to increase speech intelligibility. For patients with milder resonance disorders, therapies to reduce hypernasality and nasal emissions used in persons with cleft lip and palate are helpful. These include drills to maximize available velopharyngeal timing and closure. Lowering the habitual fundamental frequency decreases the perception of hypernasality. Speaking with a wider mouth opening can also reduce perceived hypernasality and reduce nasal emission because air, like all gases and fluids, takes the path of least resistance, directing speech air and energy through the mouth rather than through the nose.

Articulatory Valve

At the articulatory valve, the airstream and energy coming from the larynx are shaped into speech sounds. The articulators create valves in the oral cavity where the airstream is shaped in several ways. First, air and acoustic energy are briefly and completely blocked in the production of stop phonemes. Second, constrictions are created between articulatory sites in the production of continuant phonemes. Third, the height, front-to-back position of the tongue, and lip rounding create the acoustic characteristics of vowels. In dynamic speech, nearly 100 muscles and thousands of neurological impulses per second are required to make the articulatory adjustments for intelligible utterances.

The apraxia of speech discussed above often results in articulatory **additions** and **substitutions**. The coordination and movement dysarthrias, such as those involving the cerebellum and extrapyramidal systems, can also include the addition and substitution of speech sounds. Flaccid and spastic dysarthrias often cause omissions and distortions. According to Duffy (1995), in unilateral upper motor neuron dysarthria "The most common deviant speech characteristics are imprecise articulation and irregular articulatory breakdowns, both of which may be apparent during contextual speech and AMRs [alternate motion rates]" (p. 232).

Paralysis of the tongue primarily causes articulatory **distortions** and **omissions**. Spasticity, such as seen in cerebral palsy, as well as flaccidity of extrinsic and intrinsic tongue muscles, result in **reduced range of motion** for shaping the airstream into speech sounds. Spasticity and flaccidity also affect the rate of movement of the tongue and other articulators, contributing to distorted and imprecise speech sound production. In addition, ataxia and hypokinesia cause slow, sluggish movements of the tongue and other articulators. Generally, paralysis of the muscles necessary to elevate the tip of the tongue causes the most articulatory disruptions. Muscle rigidity, including the **masked face** seen in some patients with Parkinson's disease, also impairs overall facial muscle movements and contributes to articulatory distortions and omissions.

Dysarthrias affecting the articulatory valve can cause unintelligible speech. **Intelligibility** is the ability to be understood and is usually measured as a percentage. For example, a patient is said to be 25%, 50%, or 90% intelligible. Improving speech intelligibility is a primary goal in dysarthria therapies because of the role functional communication plays in a patient's quality of life.

Several therapies focusing on the articulatory valve can improve a patient's speech intelligibility (Tanner, 1999a). As described more fully below, slowing the rate of speech improves intelligibility by compensating for the sluggish movements of the articulators and allowing them to approach their ideal articulatory points of contact in dynamic speech. Speech intelligibility can also be improved by exaggerating individual sounds. Therapies for individual phonemes include muscle strengthing, range-of-motion drills, and precision and coordination exercises.

Dysarthria and Prosodic Disturbances

To various degrees, all of the dysarthrias impair speech prosody, and ataxic dysarthria is fundamentally a prosodic disorder. Speech prosody, defined most broadly, includes pitch, loudness, and quality of voice in addition to speech rate and fluency. Consequently, any neuromuscular disorder affecting phoneme precision, voice quality, rate of speech, and stress-intonation, either directly or indirectly, is a prosodic disturbance. Therapies for dysarthria often require slowing the patient's rate of speech and syllable-by-syllable speech production. As a result, dysarthria and the treatments for it may disrupt the patient's prosody.

Multiple and Mixed Dysarthrias

It is common for two or more dysarthrias to occur in the same patient at the same time or for one dysarthria to evolve into another during the course of an illness. Duffy (1995) reports that 34.7% of all dysarthrias and 31.6% of all motor speech disorders seen in the speech pathology section at the Mayo Clinic (Rochester) from 1987 to 1990 were of the mixed variety. Spastic, flaccid, and ataxic dysarthrias were the most common single types encountered. Hypokinetic dysarthria was the fourth most common single variety, followed by hyperkinetic dysarthria. "A combination of two dysarthrias represented 84% of all cases of mixed dysarthrias, 14% contained three dysarthria types, and 2% contained a combination of four types" (Duffy, 1995, p. 241).

Classifying motor speech disorders by the level of neurological impairment, rather than listing and describing all the diseases and injuries to the brain and nervous system causing neuromuscular disorder, is a logical, scientific, and efficient method of dysarthria diagnosis and treatment. Although related, the therapies for each level of deficit have different goals, objectives, and methods. However, even classifying motor speech disorders by the level of neurological impairment has its shortcomings. The high rate of multiple and mixed dysarthrias shows that neurological diseases and injuries often impair multiple neurological systems and that rigid localization and compartmentalization of symptoms for neurological disorders are often fraught with error. Duffy (1995) notes: "Unfortunately, no rule of nature obligates neurologic disease to restrict itself to the divisions we impose upon it" (p. 234).

According to Zemlin (1998), there are 11 recognized **systems** in the human body (a system comprises two or more organs combined to exhibit a functional unity): skeletal, articular (joints and ligaments), muscular, digestive, vascular, nervous, respiratory, urinary, reproductive, endocrine (glands of the body), and integumentary (skin, hair, nails). The brain and nervous system operate holistically; no single part functions completely independently of other systems. This is particularly true during communication. "With just a moment of thought it becomes apparent that no one of these systems is independent of the others. The speech mechanism draws heavily on some systems and less heavily on others, but either directly or indirectly, it is dependent upon all of the systems of the body" (p. 30). Tetnowski (2003) comments on speech disorders and strict localization philosophies: "If we knew all there was to know about human behaviors, modern brain imaging techniques would be the sole tool required to identify the symptoms, strengths, and weaknesses of our patients with neurogenically based communication disorders" (p. ix).

Principles of Dysarthria Therapy

Duffy (1995) suggests that the primary goals of therapy for motor speech disorders are **restoration**, **compensation**, and **adjustment**. These general management goals ultimately help neurogenic patients maximize the effectiveness and efficiency of communication. However, it is unlikely that patients suffering from severe neuromuscular disorders, especially progressive ones such as amyotrophic lateral sclerosis, multiple sclerosis, and Parkinson's disease, will ever have complete restoration of normal communication abilities. "It is crucial that clinicians and patients realize that full restoration of normal speech is not a realistic treatment goal in most cases" (Duffy, 1995, p. 372).

Tanner (1999a, pp. 213–215) provides eight general dysarthria therapies for stroke patients. These therapies are applicable to dysarthria arising from most neurological injuries.

1. *Slowing the rate of speech:* In most activities, the faster an action is performed, the less precise it is, hence the old adage "Haste makes waste." This principle holds true for speaking. The faster a person talks, the less precisely each sound is made. When the rate of speech exceeds about 600 hundred words per minute, most persons become unintelligible. For many survivors of strokes, reducing the rate of speech helps them adjust for muscle weakness or paralysis of the speech system and allows them to relearn how to produce each sound clearly and precisely. In the course of rehabilitation, the patient can begin to talk progressively faster once again.

2. *Exaggerating individual sounds:* Speech can often be improved significantly by exaggerating individual sounds. Although the patient may find it difficult to get into this habit while talking, after a while it becomes natural, and the greater the exaggeration, the clearer the speech becomes.

3. *Clearly producing the final sounds of words:* In normal speech, there is a tendency to produce the first sound of a word more clearly than the sounds in the middle or at the end. When the stroke survivor with dysarthria is encouraged to produce the final sounds of a word as clearly as the first and middle sounds, speech improves, sometimes dramatically.

4. *Opening the mouth more widely:* A singer opens the mouth more widely to allow the voice to radiate more effectively. For a stroke survivor with dysarthria, it is also sometimes helpful to open the mouth more widely when speaking. This allows the patient

to produce sounds more clearly and reduce the tendency to muffle speech. It also reminds the patient to use slow speech and to exaggerate each sound.

5. *Speaking more loudly:* Speech has to be loud enough to be understood. No matter how clearly or precisely the sounds are made, speech will not be heard if it is too quiet. Sometimes having the stroke survivor sit or stand with erect posture helps increase loudness.

6. *Working on specific sounds:* For many patients with dysarthria, the sounds that occur when the tongue reaches the top of the mouth are the most difficult to make. Particularly troublesome are the sounds produced at the top and front of the mouth, such as *t, th,* and *d*. As a result, the speech-language clinician may want the patient to perform exercises to strengthen and improve the movement of the tongue. These exercises are generally speech drills, but sometimes nonspeech activities are used such as trying to touch the nose with the tongue or sticking the tongue out as far as possible. However, it is usually best to give the patient speech rather than nonspeech exercises because speech exercises transfer more naturally to speaking situations.

7. *Setting standards:* Sometimes just having the patient try harder to produce speech clearly will result in significant improvement. One way of doing this is to set up a number system that reflects the patient's increased efforts. A scale of 1 to 10 works best. On this scale, 5 represents the normal, easy, effortless way people usually speak. Number 1 is unintelligible speech produced in a slurred, distorted manner. Number 10 represents per . . . fect . . . ly . . . ar . . . tic . . . u . . . la . . . ted . . . sp . . . ee . . . ch in which every sound is made with maximum precision. Setting the goal at 8 or 9 and praising the patient for trying to reach it results in more precise speech, as well as providing a way of measuring and rewarding improvement.

8. *Other therapies:* Voice, respiratory support, nasalization, and speech rhythm are other areas that may need improvement. The patient with a stroke may be given exercises designed to have the voice box produce voice or improve the quality of the sound. Several therapies are available to patients with dysarthria who need to learn how to reduce nasal resonance or to improve the rhythm of speech.

There is a parallel between the neuromuscular therapies provided by physical therapists and speech-language pathologists. Of course, a major difference between speech and physical therapy is that the physical therapist often can physically adjust body parts. The speech-language pathologist often finds it impossible to physically move the patient's speech muscles. Therefore, creative methods of strengthing, coordinating, and positioning these muscles must be found. Nevertheless, although each dysarthria requires attention to its particular neuromuscular deficiency, and although therapy goals and objectives must address unique aspects of flaccidity, spasticity, ataxia, and so forth, the above general therapies for dysarthria can be helpful for most patients with any type of dysarthria.

The goals of compensation can involve **prosthetic devices, medications, therapies,** and **alternative means of communication.** Duffy (1995) also notes that adjustment for many patients involves ending or changing careers and making significant lifestyle changes. Unfortunately, not all patients are candidates for rehabilitation, and the goals of treatment may change from overcoming the disorder to accepting it and its implications.

In most patients with neurogenic communication disorders, psychological adjustment involves the grief response and accepting unwanted changes associated with loss of self, person, and object (Tanner, 2003d). Some progressive disorders create special conditions, so that passing through the stages of grieving may be impeded by exacerbation and remission of the physical symptoms. For example, some patients may return to denial and bargaining during periods of remission, and their progression to acceptance may be delayed.

Case Studies in Motor Speech Disorders

Case Study 6.1   A High School Wrestler with Ataxic Dysarthria

FREDDY

Freddy didn't care that varsity wrestling was not a glamorous sport like football or basketball. While hundreds of students and townspeople attended football and basketball games, only a handful came to the wrestling matches. Even the "Mat Maids," cheerleaders for the team, sometimes forgot the games. It didn't matter to Freddy because he loved the sport. Tragically, during one of the tournament games, an opponent put Freddy in a hold, pinching a blood vessel and forever changing his life.

Freddy's wrestling team had made the tournament, and for the first time, the high school bleachers were full of spectators. Freddy's parents were sitting in the front row, and he waved to them as he approached the mat. His opponent for the first round was no one special, and Freddy's coach told him that this would be an easy win. After the usual squaring off, the contest began. On the first throw-down, Freddy was placed in a hold resembling the old half-Nelson, where his head was forcibly turned to the right and the full weight of his body was placed on it. Ninety seconds into the first round, Freddy lost consciousness and the paramedics rushed to his aid. When his limp body was placed on a stretcher, loaded into an ambulance, and rushed to the hospital, everyone knew his injury was serious.

On the way to the hospital, Freddy suffered a seizure. Two doctors and several nurses met the ambulance when it arrived, and Freddy was rushed to the emergency room. A tracheotomy was performed to help his breathing, and the doctors and nurses worked for hours to save his life. Early the next morning Freddy was sent to the radiology department, and the neurologist's and emergency room physicians' suspicions were confirmed: Freddy had suffered severe brain injury.

Clinical Sidebar 6.1
A seizure is a sudden onset of symptoms, usually manifest as a series of violent spasms and body jerks. The severity of seizures can range from grand mal (generalized) to petit mal (small). Seizures result from brain damage or irregularities and can cause brain damage. What effects do seizure medications have on the patient's speech symptoms and overall arousal level? Can they impede therapy?

One or more of the arteries supplying blood to Freddy's brain had been pinched during the match. As a result, the blood supply to his brain was interrupted long enough to cause irreversible damage. The primary part of the brain damaged was the cerebellum, resulting in ataxia so severe as to render him unable to walk. Freddy's family's health insurance would not pay for the motorized wheelchair he wanted, but fortunately, the community and his friends stood by him. One evening a benefit was held for Freddy, and hundreds of persons from the community came to the high school to watch amateur comedy skits, juggling acts, musical renditions, and magic shows. Enough money was donated to purchase the expensive wheelchair Freddy wanted. At the conclusion of the program, Freddy thanked the audience in a speech that he and his speech-language pathologist had worked on for weeks.

When Freddy first heard that the benefit was being planned, he asked the clinician if they could prepare a speech to thank people for their kindness and support. The clinician agreed but was uncertain whether Freddy would be able to speak intelligibly. His severe ataxic dysarthria had resulted in distorted speech, and his intelligibility was less than 30%. However, Freddy insisted, and the goal was set. They had 3 weeks.

Freddy took the lead in writing the speech, dictated to the clinician, assuring the audience that he would approach the challenges of his injury with the same resolve that had marked his wrestling career. Once the speech was written, Freddy had to learn to speak it clearly and articulately.

Freddy's speech coordination was impaired. The damage to his cerebellum had disrupted the rate, rhythm, speed, and force of speech articulation. Freddy's respiration and voicing coordination were also impaired, causing poorly articulated speech sounds produced with irregular pitch and loudness fluctuations. Because of these motor speech deficits, most persons could not understand what he was saying.

The first goal of therapy was to reduce his rate of speech. Red lines were drawn on the written script to show him where to pause to create boundaries between words. The length of the pauses was indicated by the corresponding length of the pause lines. This helped Freddy to slow his rate of speech by increasing the number and duration of the pauses, immediately improving his intelligibility.

The second goal of therapy was to increase the precision of each phoneme. Freddy was taught to exaggerate each sound. He was shown the proper positioning for the speech sounds and how to make them. The clinician and Freddy also created a feedback system and a method of communicating goals. Speech precision was placed on a scale of 1 to 10, where 1 represented extremely imprecise speech sounds and 10 was perfect articulation. The agreed-upon goal was to try to achieve an 8 or better. The result was more effort and, consequently, improved speech precision. This therapy was used to improve consonants and vowels.

Freddy was also taught to use the appropriate amount of stress. He tended to stress syllables and words that did not need it while neglecting to emphasize those that did. On the script, he was shown where stress was appropriate and how to use the correct amount on syllables and words. Because Freddy's voice quality tended to be harsh, he was also shown how to reduce laryngeal tension.

The big day arrived, and the high school gymnasium where Freddy had been injured was full. A master of ceremonies was on hand, and door prizes were offered. The performers were ambitious, energetic, and enthusiastic, but no one would confuse them with professionals. The light-hearted event brought out the best in all who had volunteered to participate. At the evening's end, Freddy was wheeled to the platform and clearly read his prepared speech to the standing ovation of the audience.

Case Study 6.2   Alleged Medical Malpractice and Spastic Cerebral Palsy

SHANTELL JOSEPH

Shantell was not the first child born to her upper-middle-class family. There were two older children, and although her brother Ron was in special education for a mild delay in speech and language, both children were physically and mentally normal. At the first indication that she was pregnant, Shantell's mother, Elizabeth, arranged for the best prenatal care and immediately stopped drinking alcohol, including her usual glass of wine with dinner. She took pregnancy seriously and responsibly, and when the delivery went tragically wrong, she blamed the obstetrician for Shantell's spastic cerebral palsy. Years of litigation followed.

For 8 months, Elizabeth did everything she could do to ensure that Shantell would develop normally. She exercised, took vitamin and mineral supplements, ate well, and visited her physician regularly. During the final weeks of pregnancy, Elizabeth started to show signs of premature delivery, and medication was prescribed to delay the birth. Elizabeth also complied with the doctor's order that she spend most of her time lying down. The day her contractions began, the doctor promised to meet her at the hospital. This was also the day the nightmare of miscommunication and allegedly improper medical care forever changed Elizabeth's life and Shantell's future.

When the contractions began in earnest, the doctor was nowhere to be found. No one knows if her telephone order increasing the medication to delay the birth was misunderstood or if she had simply prescribed the wrong dosage and perhaps the wrong medication. Elizabeth spent many hours in the delivery room trying to postpone the delivery until the doctor arrived. However, she could not be found, and there was no other obstetrician to help with the birth. Finally, when the doctor arrived, Shantell's birth was slow and difficult due to the medication and several other unexpected complications involving the umbilical cord and placenta.

Elizabeth nearly died of blood loss, and Shantell experienced stress during birth. According to the plaintiff's expert witnesses, Shantell's brain was deprived of oxygen during the delivery. Because she could not be aroused, she was immediately given oxygen and rushed to the pediatric intensive care unit in a flaccid state. She was separated from her mother, and what should have been a time of joy and bonding was one of anxiety and fear. According to the attorneys, it was an unnecessary tragedy that better planning and communication could have prevented. When Shantell was 3 years old, her parents sued the obstetrician for medical malpractice, seeking damages and compensation for therapies and other services she would require for the rest of her life.

During the discovery phase of the trial, the attorneys representing the obstetrician asserted that motor speech disorders ran in the Joseph family. They noted that Shantell's father had been in special education as a youngster for a speech disorder and that her brother, Ron, required therapy for a motor speech disorder. The obstetrician's experts stated that Shantell suffered from verbal apraxia, a speech disorder that ran in the Joseph family. The defense attorneys wanted to show that Shantell's communication disorder was inherited to limit the obstetrician's liability. The issue became whether Shantell suffered from verbal apraxia and whether her father and brother also had this motor speech programming disorder.

As is often the case in medical malpractice trials, expert witnesses for each side provided evaluations, documents, and depositions. The first issue involved the definition of apraxia of speech. Shantell and Ron were evaluated by an independent speech-language pathologist. As the defense attorneys proposed, the evaluation showed that Ron did indeed suffer from apraxia of speech. Although the therapists treating him labeled the disorder in various ways, it involved motor conceptualizing, programming, and executing purposeful speech acts. Several research articles showing that developmental apraxia of speech has an inherited component were also submitted. The plaintiffs conceded that Shantell's brother had apraxia of speech and that there might be a genetic predisposition to it, but they stated that Shantell had spastic dysarthria and that a history of apraxia of speech in the Joseph family was irrelevant.

Shantell had classic speech symptoms of spastic dysarthria. First and most obvious symptom was spastic paraplegia. Shantell had increased bilateral muscular tone and exaggerated tendon reflexes. The neurologist's report clearly stated a diagnosis of spastic paraplegia. The speech evaluation also showed spasticity of the speech muscles, with consequent imprecise production of consonants and prosodic disturbances. In addition, Shantell's voice had a strained-strangled quality. An issue arising during discovery was whether spastic dysarthria could be considered an aspect of apraxia of speech. The defense claimed that in a broad definition of apraxia of speech, upper motor neuron damage and the resulting speech symptoms could be considered an apraxia and that Shantell's spasticity involved execution of the motor act.

Apparently, the defense ultimately decided that their case for an inherited apraxia of speech and their claim that spastic dysarthria is, in fact, an aspect of impaired motor speech programming would not convince a judge and jury. A company that determined the costs of habilitation and related expenses for

Clinical Sidebar 6.2
Spastic muscles contract excessively when they are quickly and forcefully stretched. However, when they are gradually, slowly, and gently moved, they usually do not contract forcefully in response to displacement. To train spastic speech muscles to function more normally, clinicians do not force them into position; rather, they have the patient gradually, slowly, and gently position them for speech production. What effect do spastic laryngeal muscles have on voice quality?

birth defects projected how much it would cost to care for, train, and educate Shantell throughout her life. Days before the case went to trial, the parties settled out of court. Although the attorneys did not disclose the terms of the settlement, the parties to the case were told that Shantell would receive the care she required.

Case Study **6.3**   Cerebral Palsy and Clavicular Breathing

KAREN LUFKIN

People talk about the courage and resolve of the disabled, but few understand the challenges and obstacles many of them must face in an ordinary day. When a person with severe cerebral palsy manages to attain the academic and clinical requirements to become a certified speech-language pathologist, her courage and resolve are truly remarkable. What made Karen Lufkin a remarkable person was not that she made the sacrifices that many graduate students must make, but that she made them while having to think consciously about the most basic action in life: breathing. She practiced her beloved profession for nearly three decades before death took this amazing woman from the special needs students who learned so much from her.

Karen's resolve and determination were apparent from the day she was born. By all accounts, she should never have survived the delivery, and she spent most of her first weeks in a neonatal intensive care unit. Her ability to breathe on her own was always marginal, and when she entered college to pursue a degree in speech pathology and audiology, dormitory life was not an option. Karen moved to a nursing home near the university's speech and hearing department. With the assistance of an aide, she traveled to and from her phonetics, anatomy, methods, organics, stuttering, and language courses in her wheelchair. During class, she combatted her spastic respiratory muscles with clavicular breathing, working consciously to counter the reverse abdominal breathing commonly seen in spasticity by lifting and expanding her chest using her upper thoracic and neck muscles. For several years, she pursued her dream of becoming a speech-language pathologist. Unlike most students who dream of professional accomplishments, Karen's dreams did not float through her mind in the comfort of a dorm bed.

Karen slept in an iron lung. Because of her compromised respiration, she needed it to breathe when she slept. The huge lung took up most of the space in the small nursing home room. Made of galvanized steel, it was 7 feet long and 3 feet wide and was held 4 feet from the floor by supporting structures. It weighed nearly 500 pounds. When it was operating, there was a hissing sound of air rushing in and out of the chamber, followed by a low-pitched "clunk" as the main valve closed.

Clinical Sidebar 6.3
An iron lung, also known as a *Drinker Respirator*, is a mechanical device that changes the air pressure inside a metal tube and operates on Boyle's law. When the pressure inside the tube is less than the atmospheric pressure, air flows in (inspiration). When the pressure in the tube is greater than the atmospheric pressure, air flows out (exhalation). What disease accounted for many individuals being confinement to Drinker Respirators in the mid-1900s?

Karen needed assistance to enter the iron lung. Each night, two nurses' aides lifted her from the wheelchair and placed her on a sliding table. With Karen lying on her back, the aides slid the table into the iron lung until her head was inserted in a circular rubber valve. Then the aides tightened the valve around Karen's neck until a seal was created. Next, several large locking devices were engaged and Karen's lower body was sealed from the atmosphere. One of the aides then adjusted the control panel, and the iron lung began to breathe for Karen. At regular intervals, air was pumped in and out of the lung, the frequency and extent of the pumping corresponding to Karen's resting oxygen needs. This early iron lung also had a mirror placed above Karen's face at a 45-degree angle, permitting her to see and be seen by persons standing or sitting behind her. With the help of the iron lung, Karen did not need to think about breathing.

Case Study **6.4** Apraxia of Speech Without Oral Apraxia

STEPHANIE

Stephanie took the job as a clerk in the convenience store only to save enough money to return to college and continue pursuing her degree in English. The latest round of tuition increases and the high cost of housing had forced her to drop out and take the full-time, temporary job. Now, 11 years later, Stephanie is the assistant manager of the store and a stroke survivor. She also has apraxia of speech and struggles daily to program her articulators.

Stephanie suffered from migraine headaches all of her adult life. They started when she was a teenager and occurred more frequently in her early 20s. Once, she was returning from snow sledding when a migraine came on with such intensity that she lost the ability to speak. She knew what she wanted to say but her speech muscles did not work. Stephanie's friends took her to the emergency room of the hospital, where several tests were done, including magnetic resonance imaging of her brain. The doctors prescribed several drugs to prevent migraines or decrease their severity once they began. However, one day at work, a severe migraine rendered her unable to finish her shift. An ambulance took her to the hospital, again without the ability to speak normally. This time the symptoms did not resolve spontaneously, and the doctors diagnosed a cerebrovascular accident.

After 6 days in the acute care ward, Stephanie was transferred to the rehabilitation wing for intensive speech therapy. The speech-language pathologist administered several tests to diagnose her communication disorder and to design the appropriate therapies. Although Stephanie had some word-finding difficulty in conversational speech, the main neurogenic communication disorder was apraxia of speech. She had difficulty repeating vowels and consonants in isolation. She also had problems repeating one-, two-, and three-syllable words and was able to repeat longer word combinations less than 50% of the time. When trying to speak normally, Stephanie was aware of her errors, but she was rarely able to correct the programming mistakes. She also struggled with the placement of her articulators during speech.

Clinical Sidebar 6.4
In apraxia of speech, the motor speech programming errors occur more frequently on initial and more infrequent phonemes, on longer and more infrequent words, and with more complex articulatory adjustments. A general principle of therapy for apraxia of speech is to begin with simple motor speech programming and then move gradually and systematically to more complex forms. Research has shown that apraxia of speech in patients with aphasia indicates a poor prognosis. Why?

Although apraxia of speech and oral apraxia often co-occur in cerebrovascular accidents, Stephanie's ability to program and execute nonspeech oral movements was largely intact. She could purposefully and easily program her muscles to blow air from her lungs, smile, bite her lower lip, and puff her cheeks. She had no problem pretending to purse her lips as if kissing a baby. She could voluntarily lick her lips and protrude, retract, elevate, lateralize, and depress her tongue. Her ability to make purposeful, nonspeech oral movements proved to be helpful in dealing with a nagging and persistent problem of apraxia of speech: placing her articulators properly during speech.

Stephanie was discharged from the rehabilitation unit and eventually returned to work. She also received outpatient speech therapy for her residual apraxia of speech deficits. During rehabilitation, although she regained most of the ability to purposefully program her articulators for speech production, she was frequently unable to produce the /f/ phoneme. In the hospital's rehabilitation unit, she had drilled on several difficult phonemes and was eventually able to develop the muscular programming and control necessary to produce them. For example, she had difficulty with the /g/ phoneme. With her therapist's guidance, she learned to create adequate breath support and then to expel it gradually. To get her vocal cords to vibrate on the voiced consonant, she hummed during exhalation. Then the therapist showed her the proper positioning of the articulators using photo cards and a mirror, and she practiced making the sound. Because the /g/ sound occurs in the back of the throat, out of sight, she also used several sounds to "lead into" the /g/ phoneme. By progressing from easily programmed and executed sounds to the difficult /g/, she eventually was able to produce it. However, Stephanie could not master the /f/ phoneme using these therapies.

Although the /f/ sound is produced in the front of the mouth and was easily modeled by the therapist, no amount of drilling could help Stephanie program it consistently, especially when it occurred in the initial position of words. At work, for example, when a customer asked for directions, Stephanie was unable to say clearly, "Aisle four." Because of the apraxia of speech, she said, "Aisle tufor, no, I mean, suhor, uh uh, sooor." Finally, in desperation, she held up four fingers and pointed to the aisle, suffering the customer's perplexed expressions.

In outpatient therapy, Stephanie found that if she concentrated on nonspeech oral movements before making the /f/ phoneme, she could usually produce it. She concentrated on the oral movements necessary to bite her lower lip and then produced the /f/ sound correctly. Stephanie's clinician supplied word lists with the /f/ phoneme in the initial position of words. Stephanie consciously programmed her articulators to bite her lower lip and then shift that movement to the word with the /f/ phoneme. She also learned to program this sound the same way when it occurred in the medial and final positions of words. For several years following her stroke,

Stephanie still had occasional difficulty programming the /f/ phoneme. Each time she started to struggle with it, she remembered to concentrate on biting her lower lip and then gradually program the phoneme correctly. What was once a debilitating speech disorder gradually became an occasional minor nuisance.

Case Study 6.5   Apraxia of Speech in a 52-Year-Old Newspaper Editor

CORRINE CLINE

Corrine Cline is the first adult patient with a neurogenic disorder you will evaluate alone, and after reading her chart, you seriously question your competence to do so. You are only a second-year graduate student, and your name tag reads "student clinician." Fortunately, your clinical supervisor has reminded you that most student clinicians question their competence at some time, and those who do not should. A feeling of inadequacy shows that you have the proper perspective and appreciate the magnitude of the undertaking. You will soon enter the patient's hospital room and begin the evaluation. Several weeks ago, the patient, Corrine Cline, fell ill and silent at work. According to the chart, she suffered a cerebrovascular accident and is partially paralyzed on the right side.

You enter the hospital room and see a middle-aged woman watching television. She is sitting at a small table next to the hospital bed. You introduce yourself, explain your professional role, and ask her to describe her communication disorder. Corrine does her best. Struggling to use telegraphic, forced speech, she says several times, "I know what I want to say, but I cannot say it."

You know that her statement suggests several levels of communication impairments. First, Corrine may understand the images, sensations, and intuitions in her mind but may have no words to express them—a description of expressive aphasia. Second, she may be describing not the loss of words for expression, but the motor speech programming necessary to utter them. She may have apraxia of speech (verbal apraxia). Finally, she may be describing the effects of paralysis and the resulting inability to make her speech muscles valve the compressed air coming from her lungs: dysarthria.

The first aspect of your evaluation involves testing for aphasia. You have been taught the theory and administration of several aphasia batteries. However, at this clinical site, your supervisor suggests that, rather than rely on one instrument, you should administer sections of several aphasia tests. You do so and assess the patient's ability to follow directional commands, point to objects when named, and answer "yes" and "no" correctly. You see whether Corrine can match printed and written words to pictures, read aloud, and follow written instructions. Then you have her write sentences, name objects, and write to dictation. Next, you assess her verbal ability to describe and name common objects, complete sentences, and speak spontaneously. You also test her mathematical expression and reception, because math too is a language. Based on the results of the aphasia testing, you find that the stroke has had little effect on the fabric of Corrine's language.

Testing for dysarthria includes determining Corrine's respiratory support for speech production. You check to see whether she can create the necessary breath support for speech and sustain it in a controlled, efficient manner. You also assess voice quality, onset, and control, as well as pitch range and overall loudness. You decide that when the patient can program speech motorically, it is about 90% intelligible due to the paresis of her articulatory muscles, particularly those of her tongue. Fortunately, it appears that the stroke did not interfere with her nasal valving mechanism, and she is not hypernasal. Her speech prosody is only minimally affected.

Clinical Sidebar 6.5
Some patients are so apraxic as to be unable to program the respiratory coordination necessary for speech. They cannot expel air for phonation and articulation. To provide visual feedback about airflow and speech production, a sheet of tissue paper is placed in front of the patient's mouth and the patient is encouraged to blow on it while attempting to speak. What other visual feedback methods might you use with a patient who has severe apraxia of speech?

During the testing, Corrine struggles to produce sounds, syllables, words, and phrases purposefully. Curiously, she can say some words automatically. Although this is the first patient you have evaluated with a neurogenic communication disorder, you suspect that this automatic-purposeful dichotomy in speaking is *automatic speech.* The best example of such speech occurred when Corrine repeatedly pointed to a picture of her daughter on the table, and tried to say her name: Maggie. It sounded like "aggie," "staggie," "uh-aggie," and "raggie." Then, when Corrine's attention was directed elsewhere and she gave little thought to the word, she easily and correctly said, "I can't seem to say 'Maggie' today," although with minor distortions caused by the dysarthria. You have learned that this automatic speech behavior is usually considered part of apraxia of speech. You begin this aspect of the evaluation with a clinical hypothesis that Corrine Cline's major neurogenic communication disorder is apraxia of speech.

Testing for apraxia of speech primarily involves repeating utterances of increasing length. Apparently, repeating requires the patient to program her articulators consciously, making the behavior more voluntary. First, she must repeat vowels in isolation; Corrine repeats several of them, although she struggles and has difficulty placing her articulators in the proper positions. In the "Comments" section of the test, you note that she also has problems programming airflow, creating voicing, and producing the articulatory positioning for vowels. You similarly test continuants, plosives, affricates, and diphthongs, with Corrine scoring poorly on each subtest. Testing her ability to repeat syllables of increasing length also shows severe impairment in motor programming, sequencing, and executing speech movements during repetitions. You continue to test multiple word constructions, multiple repetitions of multisyllable words, progressively longer words, and phrases. The final aspect of this test battery for apraxia of speech focuses on the patient's ability to count, say the alphabet, and name the days of the week and months of the year. Corrine continues to struggle with these tasks. On a positive note, you observe that she is usually aware of her errors; unfortunately, she is rarely self-corrective. According to her test score, Corrine suffers from severe apraxia of speech and oral apraxia. Your clinical hypothesis is confirmed: This patient's primary neurogenic communication disorder is apraxia of speech.

Case Study **6.6** A 38-Year-Old Woman with Amyotrophic Lateral Sclerosis

BARBARA

The early signs of disease were barely perceptible. Barbara was simply too busy taking care of her two children, working part-time, and dealing with her failing marriage to focus on them. The first indications Barbara could not ignore were the muscle cramping, weakness, and trembling in her hands. Even her children commented on her shaking hands during mealtime. But it was the chronic fatigue that took her to the doctor, and after a series of tests, she gave her the bad news: Barbara had Lou Gehrig's disease—amyotrophic lateral sclerosis (ALS).

Barbara met with a medical social worker and enrolled in an ALS support group. She learned that ALS occurs less frequently in women than in men, and she was relatively young to have it. ALS is a rare disease affecting about 1 in 100,000 persons. The hard reality was that she would not survive. According to the social worker, the average survival rate was about 3 years, although some patients lived for 20 years or more. There were many theories about the cause or causes of the disease, but no one knew what was causing Barbara's muscles to waste away.

Over several months, the disease progressively impaired Barbara's walking, dressing, and other activities of daily living. The occupational and physical therapists helped to slow the effects of the muscular degeneration and found ways to compensate for the functions she was gradually losing. Barbara worked hard, but her increasing fatigue and the nausea caused by her strong medications limited her participation in occupational and physical therapies.

As the disease progressed, Barbara's speech began to degenerate. At first, a few consonants were slurred, beginning with *t* and *d;* others soon followed. Barbara began to drool and constantly had to wipe her mouth. Her speech slowed and became monotonous, with no changes in pitch. Her voice became weak, raspy, and nasal. She could not create the air pressure necessary for intelligible speech due to the weak muscles and air leaking through her nose. Before Barbara completely lost her voice, she voiced all speech sounds, even the voiceless ones. This was an automatic compensatory behavior to increase loudness, but it also reduced her intelligibility. Together, Barbara and the speech-language pathologist did all they could to stave off the speech degeneration, but over several months it progressed relentlessly.

ALS is a devastating disease, not only physically but also psychologically. At first, when she began to lose her speech, she was intelligible. She could express her fears, anxiety, hopes, and resolve to defeat this terrible disease. She could tell her children that all would be well, discuss with her husband their care should she die, and participate in her church. Early in the course of the disease, speech served powerful psychological functions. But during the middle and final stages of the disease, she lost the ability to speak at a time when she most needed to reach out to others.

The social worker and members of the support group told Barbara's family that she was likely experiencing preparatory grief—she was preparing to be separated from all the things and persons she loved. And although her marriage had been in trouble before the onset of the disease, when she lost the ability to speak all hope of reconciliation was lost. In the final stages of the disease, Barbara was even removed from the comforts of her home and placed in a nursing home for the care she required.

The social worker and members of the support group understood the stages of grieving Barbara would experience to achieve ultimate acceptance of the inevitable. At first, she denied that something was seriously wrong and postponed going to the doctor. When the test results appeared, she said that they referred to someone else. At times during the early stages, she returned to the comfort of denial; this was easy, since there were periods when she felt relatively normal. Soon, however, denial gave way to anger and bargaining, marking Barbara's frustration with this insidious and pernicious disease.

For a time, Barbara was angry at the disease, herself, her husband, her children, and even God. The frustration of dealing with the slow loss of everything she loved made her angry at the world. Through no fault of her own, she was forced to deal with this devastating disease and the pain and suffering associated with it. As often happens when people cannot defeat an all-powerful foe, she bargained with God, praying and offering future good work and a life of dedication to the church if she was spared. She tried several unorthodox medications, therapies, and treatments to gain more time to be with her young children. But the anger and bargaining did nothing to stop the disease, and Barbara became depressed. Saturated with the sad realities of the disease, she became lethargic, hopeless, and helpless.

Toward the end, the depression gradually lifted, and Barbara accepted what had happened. Her negative emotions finally dissipated, and she felt neither good nor bad. What is most important, Barbara found herself reveling in the good things that had happened to her rather than being saddened by the coming end of her life.

Clinical Sidebar 6.6
Many of the psychological symptoms caused by brain injury are similar to the psychological reactions seen in persons with functional emotional disturbances. Do you think chemical imbalances always cause severe psychological disturbances? If not, what other factors might be responsible?

SUMMARY

Motor speech disorders impair the ability to program, sequence, and execute the neuromuscular movements necessary for speech production. They affect, to varying degrees, respiration, phonation-resonance, articulation, and prosody. Apraxia of speech disrupts or eliminates the ability to program speech movements and interferes primarily with articulation. Therapies exist for apraxia of speech and for the aspects of motor speech disrupted by the dysarthrias. In addition, general therapies are available for motor speech disorders regardless of which motor system is impaired. Most patients with motor speech disorders can improve their speech precision and intelligibility, but full restoration of communication abilities is not always possible.

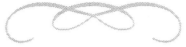

Study and Discussion Questions

1. How are motor speech disorders classified? What are the symbolic and nonsymbolic disorders?

2. Compare and contrast aphasia and apraxia of speech.

3. Describe the symptoms of apraxia of speech. How does awareness of speech errors and the ability to self-correct affect them?

4. Describe the effects of dysarthria and apraxia of speech on respiration.

5. Describe the effects of dysarthria and apraxia of speech on phonation-resonance.

6. Describe the effects of dysarthria and apraxia of speech on articulation.

7. Describe the effects of dysarthria and apraxia of speech on speech prosody.

8. List and discuss the therapies for apraxia of speech.

9. List and discuss the general principles of dysarthria therapy.

10. Compare and contrast oral apraxia and apraxia of speech.

Recommended Reading

Darley, F., Aronson, A., & Brown, J. (1975). *Motor speech disorders*. Philadelphia: Saunders.

    This is the classic textbook on motor speech disorders and categorizes them by the level of neurological involvement.

Duffy, J. (1995). *Motor speech disorders*. St. Louis: Mosby.

    Many graduate programs use this textbook in courses on apraxia of speech and the dysarthrias.

Tanner, D. (1999). *The family guide to surviving stroke and communication disorders*. Austin: PRO-ED.

    This book, written for family members of stroke victims, addresses motor speech disorders including rehabilitation (Chapters 3 and 11).

Tanner, D. (2003). Eclectic perspectives on the psychology of aphasia. *Journal of Allied Health, 32*, 256–260.

    This article examines three factors associated with the psychological adjustment to neurogenic communication disorders: organic factors, coping styles and defense mechanisms, and the response to loss.

CHAPTER SEVEN

Dysphagia

There is no love sincerer than the love of food.

George Bernard Shaw

Chapter Preview: This chapter deals with dysphagia, or swallowing disorders. Dysphagia frequently occurs with communication disorders, and speech-language pathologists have assumed primary responsibility for its diagnosis and treatment. In this chapter, dysphagia is broadly defined, and the anatomy and physiology of swallowing are discussed. The relationship of speech production and swallowing is reviewed, and the stages of a normal swallow are described. There is a review of clinical/beside screening and instrumental evaluation procedures. Case studies of dysphagia and medical malpractice litigation, as well as a description of a video swallow study, are presented. There are also cases involving a tracheotomy tube, partial glossectomy, and an unusual instance of isolated dysphagia.

OVERVIEW OF DYSPHAGIA

"It is the position of the American Speech-Language-Hearing Association (ASHA) that speech-language pathologists play a primary role in the evaluation and treatment of infants, children, and adults with swallowing and feeding disorders" (ASHA, 2001, p. III-1). Although **dysphagia** is not a communication disorder per se, speech-language pathologists have taken the lead in its diagnosis and treatment. This is natural given their education and broad knowledge of the oral-pharyngeal-laryngeal mechanism.

According to Spahr and Malone (1998), approximately 15 million Americans have a swallowing disorder. Although dysphagia can appear at any age, it occurs much more often among the elderly, particularly in nursing home patients. Young children with birth defects, pervasive developmental disorders, and neuromuscular disorders are also at higher risk for dysphagia. Incidence figures for dysphagia also depend on the researcher's definition of the disorder. Some define dysphagia narrowly as the inability to move a liquid or food substance from the mouth to the stomach. In this definition, only the motor acts of sucking, chewing, and swallowing are included. Other researchers define dysphagia broadly, including the sensory, perceptual, and cognitive awareness of the patient and his or her ability to fulfill hydration and nutritional needs orally.

In this book, a broad definition of dysphagia is used to accommodate the complexity of the disorder. In addition, broad definitions of dysphagia are often used for **forensic purposes** and during **litigation**:

> **Dysphagia:** Impairment of the emotional, cognitive, sensory, and/or motor acts involved with transferring a substance from the mouth to stomach, resulting in failure to maintain hydration and nutrition, and posing a risk of choking and aspiration. (Tanner, 2003b, p. 70)

In this definition of dysphagia, the patient's awareness and cognitive abilities are addressed relative to eating and swallowing. The patient's sensory abilities, including responses to food odors, are also considered, as well as the motor acts of moving food and liquid from the mouth to the stomach.

Relationship of Speech and Swallowing

There is a fundamental relationship between speech production and **deglutition** (swallowing). Humans are **omnivorous** and can suck, bite, tear, chew, and swallow many types of food. Over millions of years, they have developed the structures, neurology, and musculature to ingest a variety of meats, fruits, nuts, vegetables, and liquids of differing viscosity to sustain life. Human teeth can tear and grind. The lips close and seal the oral cavity to create the negative intraoral air pressure necessary for sucking. The tongue is capable of assuming the many shapes and movements necessary to move food and liquid to the posterior oral cavity in preparation for swallowing. The vocal cords reflexively close and protect the air passageway to the lungs during the swallow. The anatomical structures, neurology, and musculature necessary for these actions have evolved to permit the complex acts of sucking, chewing, and swallowing. Speech has also evolved as an **overlaid function** to deglutition; the same muscles and structures used for swallowing also are used to produce speech sounds. For example, the teeth are used for dental phonemes, the lips for plosives, and the vocal cords to produce voiced speech sounds.

Normal Swallowing

Swallowing consists of three interconnected phases: **oral, pharyngeal,** and **laryngeal-esophageal**. During eating, swallowing can occur as often as 300 times per hour (Zemlin, 1998). The oral phase, sometimes called the **buccal phase**, has two stages: **oral preparation** and **transportation**. During the preparation stage, food is **masticated** (chewed) and liquid is contained. The lips, cheeks, and jaw muscles are important in mastication. In oral preparation, a **bolus** is created by rolling the food into a ball and saturating it with liquid from the meal and saliva. During the transportation stage, the tongue moves the liquid and bolus to the back of the oral cavity in preparation for swallowing.

During the pharyngeal phase of swallowing the velum elevates, closing off the passageway to the nasal cavity. The vocal cords close to prevent the liquid and food particles from entering the lungs. In this phase, the larynx elevates and moves anteriorly, and

Table 7.1 Neurology of the Swallow

Stage/Function	Nerve	Muscle/Tissue
Oral stage (mastication)	Trigeminal (V), hypoglossal (XII), ansa cervicalis (C_1-C_2), vagus (X)	Temporalis, masseter, medial pterygoid, lateral pterygoid Intrinsic and extrinsic tongue muscles, palatoglossus
Pharyngeal stage	Glossopharyngeal (IX), vagus (X), trigeminal (V), V(3), VII, C_1-C_2	Stylopharyngeus palate, pharynx, and larynx; tensor veli palatini; hyoid and larynx
Laryngeal-esophageal stage (completion of swallow)	Facial (VII), trigeminal (V), vagus (X)	Opening of cricopharyngeus; peristalsis
Sensation: tongue	Lingual, trigeminal, chorda tympani, facial (VII), glossopharyngeal (IX)	General sensation: anterior two-thirds of the tongue Taste: anterior two-thirds of the tongue Taste and General Sensation: posterior one-third of the tongue
Oral tract	Glossopharyngeal (IX), vagus (X)	Pharynx, larynx, viscera

Sources: Arvedson and Brodsky (2002); Bass (1997); Perlman and Christensen (1997); Zemlin (1998).

the epiglottis snaps down to further protect the lungs. The tongue pistons the liquid or food mass posteriorly, and the third phase is triggered: the laryngeal-esophageal phase. In this book, the final phase is called *laryngeal-esophageal* rather than *esophageal* to emphasize the importance of the protective laryngeal actions during the combined phases and also to account for respiratory clearing actions such as throat clearing and productive coughing.

Perlman and Christensen (1997) suggest the term *pharyngealolaryngeal* to include the laryngeal activities. Table 7.1 shows the stage, function, nerve, muscle, and tissue for each phase of the swallow.

Taking food into the mouth, creating a bolus, moving it to the back of the oral cavity, and swallowing it are dynamic interconnected acts performed, for the most part, without conscious thought. Also, conversational speech frequently occurs during meals and while chewing and swallowing. Figure 7.1 shows bolus creation and movement through the oral, pharyngeal, and laryngeal-esophageal phases.

Dysphagia Evaluation

There are two separate but related aspects to a swallowing evaluation: **clinical/bedside screening** and **instrumental assessment**. Before either is completed, the patient's medical and social history is reviewed. This review includes a careful study of the patient's chart and questioning of the intake nurse or another informed party. Review of the patient's medical

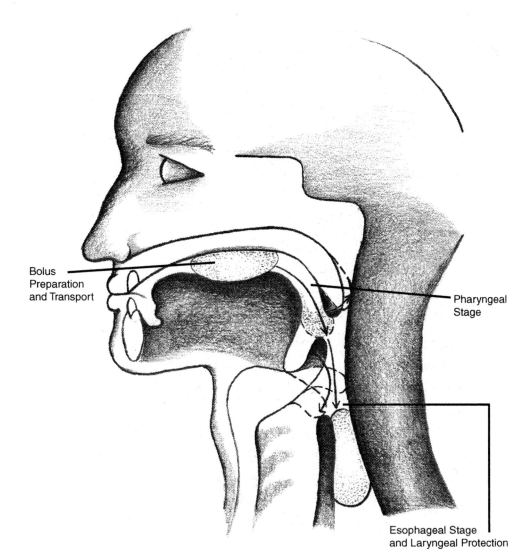

Bolus
Preparation
and Transport

Pharyngeal
Stage

Esophageal Stage
and Laryngeal Protection

Figure 7.1 Three stages of the swallow.

history reveals the admitting diagnosis. The admitting diagnosis and the report show whether the patient has a history of eating or swallowing problems. If the admitting diagnosis includes terms such as *dysphagia, dehydration, eating difficulties, swallowing problems, failure to thrive, aspiration pneumonia,* and so forth, the dysphagia evaluation usually includes a **video swallow study**. (See the section Instrumental Dysphagia Diagnostics for a detailed discussion of this radiographic procedure.) Admission with a previous diagnosis of swallowing impairments usually warrants an instrumental assessment, although a bedside screening may also be conducted. Review of the patient's medical history also provides information about disorders that compromise the patient's respiration, such as chronic obstructive pulmonary disease, emphysema, and pneumonia. The review includes previously diagnosed speech pathologies, including laryngeal dysfunctions that may impair the vocal folds' protective functioning during the swallow. It also provides information about the patient's general cognitive functioning and use of medications affecting awareness, saliva creation, and motor control.

In the clinical/bedside evaluation, the patient's swallowing normalcy or functionality during the three swallowing phases is checked. This can be scored by using a modified Likert scale, where normalcy or functionality is listed as a numerical range (Tanner & Culbertson, 1999a). For patients who are **NPO** (nothing to be given to them orally), their behaviors are assessed indirectly by observing their oral-motor functioning. If the patient is receiving food and liquids orally, the best time to do the clinical/bedside evaluation is during mealtime. In the oral phase, the patient's ability to accept food, masticate, and create a bolus is assessed. For liquids, lip seal and containment are also observed. Food and liquid transportation to the posterior oral cavity is assessed, and observations are made about impulsively and **pocketing**, in which the patient places the bolus or particles of food in the cheek and neglects to clear them.

In the pharyngeal phase, the clinician determines whether the patient can initiate the swallow purposefully and automatically. **Velopharyngeal competence** is tested by having the patient say "ah" and observing the movement of the soft palate and pharyngeal walls. The **gag reflex** is tested by gently placing a tongue blade to the posterior region of the oral cavity. The gag reflex provides information about the patient's oral sensory and motor status. At this stage, **pharyngeal peristalsis**, in which the bolus is rhythmically moved by a squeezing motion of muscles, is initiated and coordinated with other swallowing phases.

In the laryngeal-esophageal stage, assessment involves how well the patient protects the airway during the swallow and the final movement of the liquid or bolus to the stomach. Velopharyngeal closure, laryngeal elevation, and vocal cord closure are maintained, and the epiglottis covers the glottis as a protective reflex. Many of these functions cannot be observed during the clinical/bedside evaluation, but information can be obtained by observing voice quality changes, throat clearing, laryngeal elevation, and whether the patient has a productive cough.

The clinical/bedside evaluation has many limitations in detecting the safety and completeness of a swallow. This is particularly true of **silent aspiration**, in which the patient aspirates without coughing, gagging, or showing other signs that food or liquid has penetrated the lower airways. With the clinical/bedside evaluation, there is always the risk of **false positives** and **false negatives**. A false positive indicates that the patient has dysphagia when, in fact, he or she swallows normally; a false negative suggests the opposite. False positives and false negatives can also occur with instrumental assessments, but the likelihood of error is not as great.

Daniels, McAdams, Brailey, and Foundas (1997) found several factors predicting the severity of dysphagia and the need for instrumental assessment: dysphonia, dysarthria, abnormal volitional cough, abnormal gag reflex, abnormal cough reflex, cough after swallow, and voice change. Based on cases involving dysphagia and medical malpractice litigation, it is suggested that an instrumental swallowing evaluation be routinely conducted.

> The clinical practice of artificially separating swallowing into as many as four independent and distinct stages, i.e., oral preparation, transportation, pharyngeal, and laryngeal-esophageal, is misleading regarding the actual nature of chewing and swallowing. These are artificial clinical distinctions used to evaluate the swallow, show the need for radiologic evaluation, and for therapy purposes. The reality is that people put food in their mouths, chew, and then they swallow it. Artificially dividing swallowing into several independent movements is analogous to viewing running as many independent movements. For example, swallowing, as with running, cannot be completed by any of the acts occurring independently. Running and swallowing are dynamic acts. When evaluating swallowing, the bedside examination can only determine "possible" structural, neurological, or muscular deficiencies that may interfere with the movement of the bolus or liquid. There can be no certainty that a patient will or will not choke or aspirate at any level or stage based on clinical/bedside swallowing examination. If there is sufficient reason to believe that a patient has compromised swallowing, regardless of the deficient stage, the prudent clinical course is to conduct one or more instrumental evaluations of the sequentially occurring swallow. Neglecting to conduct an instrumental evaluation of the swallow in cases of suspected dysphagia is analogous to refusing to X-ray a leg for suspected fractures. (Tanner, 2003b, p. 86)

Instrumental Dysphagia Diagnostics

Several instruments can be used for dysphagia evaluations, and new ones such as **endoscopic** and **ultrasound** procedures show promise. Currently, the primary instrumental procedure is **fluoroscopy** performed as part of a video swallow study. A video swallow study is conducted in the radiology department of the medical facility. The speech-language pathologist is present when the patient swallows the **barium** liquid or paste. The real-time image of the patient's oral, pharyngeal, and laryngeal-esophageal movement of the barium is observed, and the clinician instructs the patient how to improve the swallow. Valuable information about the integrity of the swallow is obtained in addition to the patient's success in modifying deficient aspects of it. Behaviors that can reduce or eliminate barium aspiration include turning the patient's head to the affected side for vocal cord paralysis and positioning the body to maximize the effects of gravity during the swallow. Sometimes patients can reduce or eliminate aspiration by *dry swallows,* in which they repeatedly swallow without placing additional barium in their mouths. For some patients, forcefully producing a vowel at the conclusion of the swallow, and before inhalation, can help clear the air passages. When these and other behaviors are completed during the video swallow study, the clinician can determine their success and incorporate them in dysphagia therapy.

As mentioned above, procedures such as clinical/bedside screening can produce false positives and false negatives. Some patients are anxious about the video swallow study and do not perform optimally; for other patients, the procedure creates artificial situations providing unnatural results. In addition, patients' neuromuscular abilities are rarely constant and static; some patients have progressive disorders, and others achieve spontaneous recovery. Because of this variability, the clinician should be cautious in interpreting the results of the clinical/bedside and instrumental tests of dysphagia. These procedures are not exact, nor are they always reliable and valid. Repeated clinical/bedside and instrumental dysphagia evaluations are often required.

Nasogastric, Gastric, and Tracheotomy Tubes

A **nasogastric** (NG) tube is placed through the patient's nose into the stomach. It is a temporary way of providing the patient with nutritional supplements and liquids. Patients sometimes receive dysphagia therapy while the NG tube is in place. Although there are no research studies about the effects of an NG tube on the patient's swallow, it probably creates a foreign body sensation and interferes with swallowing movements. Some patients require gastrotomy, the creation of an opening directly into the stomach (Dirckx, 2001). A **gastric** tube is placed directly into the stomach in patients with dysphagia who have a poor prognosis, and nutritional supplements and liquid are given by bypassing the oral-pharyngeal-esophageal route.

A **tracheotomy** tube is placed in the patient's neck below the vocal cords. It provides a direct opening that allows air to enter the lungs and bypass the larynx and upper air passageways, and is used for patients whose respiration is compromised. When the tracheotomy tube's cuff, a balloon-like device surrounding the lower part of the tube, is inflated, food and liquid are usually prevented from entering the lungs. Some tracheotomy tubes are **fenestrated** (i.e., have windows cut into them), allowing the patient to produce voice. Tracheotomy tubes reduce laryngeal elevation and can interfere with the swallow.

Dysphagia in Geriatric and Pediatric Populations

The very old and very young are often **high-risk populations** for dysphagia and related complications. In elderly patients with dementia, dysphagia can be difficult to diagnose and treat. Because of dementia-related symptoms such as memory loss, agitation, impulsiveness, generalized intellectual deficits, and so forth, these patients present special challenges during clinical/bedside and instrumental diagnosis, and they may be unable to participate fully in dysphagia therapies. According to Cefalu (1999), high risk patients with dementia suspected of having dysphagia include those with significant weight loss or feeding difficulties, those requiring assistance with feeding, those significantly below ideal body weight, and those with concurrent depression or a history of cerebrovascular accidents.

Children with dysphagia are seen by speech-language pathologists in medical and educational settings. In young children, dysphagia diagnosis and treatment are complicated by their anatomical differences. The size, dimension, and movement differences of the oral-laryngeal structures in infants and young children are important considerations. Dysphagia associated with cleft lip and palate is unique to children. Indications for pediatric swallowing evaluations include failure to thrive, dehydration, frequent choking, significant weight loss, and apnea during feeding. Perhaps the best indication that a dysphagia evaluation needs to be conducted is the mother's report of her child's sucking, swallowing, or feeding difficulties.

Dysphagia Therapy

Patients with dysphagia are usually highly motivated to participate in therapy because re-learning to eat normally is both a drive and a reward. Clinical experience has shown that dysphagia therapy is usually successful, with most patients ultimately able to meet all or part of their hydration and nutritional needs orally. Patients with a poor prognosis are those with dementia, severe traumatic brain injury, and global aphasia.

Dysphagia therapies consist of commonsense changes in diet and modifications of chewing and swallowing behaviors. They can be separated into intervention procedures for **oral intake**, **mastication**, **transportation**, and **swallowing** deficits. Using the broad definition of dysphagia, oral intake problems can include the patient's desire to eat, impulsiveness, response to the smell of food, and recognition of liquids, food items, utensils, and other items. Therapies include counseling, instruction, and behavior modification, often in conjunction with neuropsychologists, occupational therapists, and other health care professionals.

To masticate properly, patients must have the proper dentition, jaw, and tongue mobility. When dentition is insufficient for mastication, the clinician instructs the dietary department to provide meals as liquids, pureed, chopped to various textures, or in soft form. Behavior management and instruction are provided to improve tongue mobility in creating a bolus, managing liquids, and clearing the oral cavity after chewing and swallowing are completed. Patients are also shown how to remove pocketed food from the cheeks. Properly selected patients can be trained to create a bolus and move it posteriorly prior to swallowing using bread or similar soft, manageable food. The patient can monitor liquid containment and movement by using hot or cold substances to enhance the oral sensation.

Patients with dysphagia are instructed, counseled, and trained to time the swallow correctly and to be more conscious of it. The temperature and texture of foods and the consistency of liquids can be adjusted to facilitate the swallow reflex. **Tepid foods** and **thin liquids** are usually avoided because they are more difficult to sense and manage. As stated previously, for the patient with laryngeal paralysis, **turning the head to the affected side** promotes the vocal cords' protective actions. Some patients benefit from **body positioning** to maximize the effects of gravity during the swallow. **Dry swallowing** helps some patients clear food and liquids. Certain patients find it useful to produce a **voiced phoneme** loudly after the swallow to clear the air passageways. It is helpful for some patients to take **deep breaths** before swallowing to provide air support for clearing liquids and dislodging food from the air passageways. **Oral-motor muscular strengthening exercise** may be beneficial and can be incorporated into speech therapy when appropriate. **Throat-clearing** exercises and activities to improve productive coughing are also helpful in reducing the negative effects of aspiration.

For patients who have difficulty relearning the various phases of swallowing, repeated video swallow studies may provide additional therapies that may be of benefit. Even after patients appear to have mastered safe swallowing, they should be monitored for aspiration and choking risks. For home health patients and those being discharged home, family instruction and counseling are also necessary.

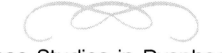

Case Studies in Dysphagia

Case Study 7.1 Litigation Regarding the Misdiagnosis of Dysphagia in a 72-Year-Old Man

ALBERT ANDERSON

Martin, the plaintiff's attorney, walked toward the jury box and began the summation. The four men and eight women would deliberate for hours, and possibly days, to reach a verdict about the death of Albert Anderson. After 2 weeks of trial and nearly 3 years of preparation, they would decide how much money, if any, the doctor, nursing home, and therapist should pay his family for the loss of their beloved father, brother, and husband. The attorney, who specialized in medical malpractice law, knew that the summation was the concluding and an important part of his presentation to the jury. He began the summation with a review of the plaintiff's case.

"During the past two weeks, we have provided you with a time line of events that led to the death of Albert Anderson. We have clearly shown that the untimely and tragic death of Mr. Anderson was the result of an uncaring and arrogant nursing home, a physician who did not keep current on postsurgical care of his patient, and a speech therapist who performed a swallowing evaluation that was below the standards of her profession." "Soon," Martin continued, "you will be required to make the important decisions about this case. You will decide whether the nursing home, doctor, and therapist were negligent in their professional conduct, and whether there is a preponderance of evidence that their behaviors led to his death. If you believe the evidence and testimony we have presented, you will also be required to determine the monetary amount to be awarded the family." Martin then placed his hands on the railing of the jury box and said in a soft voice, "Of course, the monetary judgment will not return Mr. Anderson to the living, nor will it fill the void of his passing for his family. If any good is to come from this trial, the award will likely prevent future sloppy medical decisions and perhaps spare the lives of other patients. It will also be a small symbol for the family to help them resolve their grief."

The court room was silent as Martin continued his summation. "Palo Verde Eldercare, the nursing home that professed to have the skill and ability to care for Mr. Anderson, is guilty of neglect that directly contributed to his wrongful death. We have shown that the doctors, nurses, therapists, and aides, although well intentioned, were too busy to take care of Mr. Anderson's special dietary needs. There were too few medical professionals, with too little training in dysphagia, and poor communication among them. Mr. Anderson displayed many of the signs of dysphagia: a gurgle in his chest, spiked temperature, anxiety associated with eating, dramatic weight loss, and even an X-ray showing infiltrates in his lungs. Several times,

Clinical Sidebar 7.1
Health care providers sometimes wrongly assume that because a patient does not cough or choke on food or liquid, the swallowing ability must be intact. Some patients have silent aspiration without coughing or choking. When persons choke and say that the food or liquid "went down the wrong tube," to what tube are they referring? What tube is the right one?

his daughter told the authorities that her father's ability to eat was impaired. Yet, for several months, not one medical professional associated with the nursing home saw fit to inform his doctor. He was fed a regular diet that was clearly inappropriate for him, and no one saw the signs that deadly bacteria-laden food particles were being aspirated. They even ignored his allergy to milk products. Because of the nursing home's desire for profit, it did not provide an adequate number of professionals, a protocol for proper communication among them, and proper inservice training about dysphagia and related eating disorders. The nursing home gladly accepted Mr. Anderson's money for his care but not the responsibility for his swallowing disorder."

Martin then pointed to the physician sitting at the defense table. "This doctor is one of the best heart surgeons in the Southwest. His skilled hands saved Mr. Anderson's life with the bypass surgery. He is a well-trained and skilled health care provider, deserving of respect and a respectable income. But people make mistakes, and when physicians make them, they can be deadly. For all of the doctor's surgical skills, he did not stay informed about Mr. Anderson's postsurgical recovery. He was negligent in scheduling outpatient office visits. He was negligent in communicating with the nursing staff and Mr. Anderson's family. He was negligent in not taking the time to investigate Mr. Anderson's dysphagia symptoms even when they were reported to him on several occasions. And when the doctor finally got around to investigating Mr. Anderson's dysphagia, he committed the most negligent omission: he ordered an upper GI rather than the proper video swallow study. The doctor simply did not take the time, nor did he have the training, to manage Mr. Anderson's dysphagia."

Then Martin summarized the alleged medical malpractice of the speech-language pathologist. "The speech-language pathologist was also negligent in her evaluation when the order finally was written. When she got the referral on Mr. Anderson, she did a bedside screening, missed many important symptoms of dysphagia, and, most important, did not recommend a video swallow study. She wrote in the chart and reported to the nurses that several of the patient's behaviors were 'within normal limits' when, in fact, she should have written and reported that she was 'unable to test' them. It is true that the order given to her was vague about whether to do a speech and language evaluation or a dysphagia evaluation. It is true that staff cutbacks had her doing the work of three clinicians. It is true that during the evaluation, Mr. Anderson may have had a particularly good day with eating and swallowing. All of these seem like good excuses for missing Mr. Anderson's dysphagia, but the real truth is that there was no excuse for her not performing to the level expected by the American Speech-Language-Hearing Association. There was no excuse for her not performing to the standards of professional conduct that others in her profession must meet."

Martin apologized for how nasty the trial had become and said he appreciated that the jury might have sympathy for the defendants. He said he too had sympathy for them. However, he also had sympathy for Mr. Anderson's family. And although Albert Anderson could not be present to testify in his own behalf, Martin said that the jury had an obligation to him that far exceeded the sympathy they might have for the defendants. Albert Anderson trusted the medical establishment to provide the level of care he required and assumed that all of the professionals would perform to reasonable professional standards. "What you must decide is whether Albert Anderson was properly treated for his dysphagia, and a just verdict can only be for the plaintiffs. We have clearly shown that the nursing home, doctor, and therapist, for whatever reasons, did not perform to the levels expected of them, and their malpractice directly caused the premature demise of Mr. Albert Anderson." Martin concluded the summation with a plea to the jury: "You owe it to the memory of Mr. Anderson, to his family, and to future patients with dysphagia to do the right thing. You must find for the plaintiffs and award the punitive damages that will help prevent future medical travesties like the one that resulted in the death of Mr. Albert Anderson."

Case Study 7.2   Dysphagia and Gastric Tube Placement in a 92-Year-Old Woman

FRENCHY

Her name is Audrey, but because of her French accent, the people in the nursing home simply call her Frenchy. She immigrated to the United States when she was a teenager. She spent most of her life in New Mexico, where she finally retired from the nursing profession. After suffering a stroke that robbed her of communication and left her with global aphasia, she was placed in a nursing home. Soon afterward, she began to lose weight and seemed to lose interest in life. A dysphagia evaluation was ordered.

The speech-language pathologist enters the patient's room and greets her with a smile and a left-handed shake of her hand. Frenchy acknowledges the clinician's presence by returning the smile and saying, "Tula." Frenchy remembers the clinician from previous visits when her communication abilities were evaluated. After making small talk, the clinician tells her that the purpose of the visit is to evaluate Frenchy's swallowing abilities. This is done using speech, gestures, modeling, and pictures. Frenchy appears to understand the purpose of the visit and indicates nonverbally that she will cooperate.

The clinical/bedside screening is quick and to the point. Because of Frenchy's communication problem, the clinician does a cursory oral-facial evaluation. She notes that since her last visit 2 weeks ago, the patient has developed a right facial sag, her tongue deviates to the right on protrusion, and she drools. The therapist leaves the patient's room and goes to the nurses' station. Calling the attending physician, she reports that a video swallowing study will be necessary. Both clinicians agree that this procedure will be expensive because the patient must be transferred to a nearby hospital. They also agree that it is necessary.

The next morning, an ambulance takes Frenchy to the hospital. The clinician arrives a few minutes later, and soon the patient is positioned for the procedure. She is physically able to sit upright in the specially designed chair. The radiologist and a technician enter the room and explain to Frenchy what will happen during the study. Frenchy is more than a little frightened when everyone but she dons a lead apron.

The monitor is located above and to the right of Frenchy. A blank videocassette is placed in the recorder below it for a review of the procedure if necessary. The clinician tells Frenchy to drink the white, chalky barium liquid. Frenchy, still nervous but cooperative, drinks it. The swallow is observed on the monitor as it moves from her lips to the back of her oral cavity and then down her throat. Most of the barium goes down the esophagus and, at first glance, the swallow appears successful. On closer inspection, barium is seen to pool on the vocal cords. When Frenchy inhales, it is sucked into her lungs. The patient makes no attempt to clear her throat or to cough

Clinical Sidebar 7.2
Although liquid can pool at any level of the swallowing mechanism, this usually occurs in the pyriform sinuses of the vocal folds or the vallecula at the base of the tongue. Why are hot or cold liquids and foods easier for some patients to monitor during the swallow?

the liquid out of her lungs. Because of Frenchy's global aphasia, she is unable to follow instructions about dry swallowing, clearing her throat, head and body positioning, and other therapies to help the swallow.

Frenchy is given a second opportunity to swallow the barium liquid, but this time with a thicker consistency. Most of it is propelled down her esophagus, but there is still pooling at the vocal cords, and this time, at the base of the tongue as well. Frenchy appears oblivious to the substance in her respiratory tract, and when she inhales, much of it is aspirated. Because of her communication disorder, she cannot understand instructions and alter her swallowing patterns. The radiologist, technician, and speech-language pathologist agree that Frenchy has failed the swallowing study.

That afternoon, the physician and speech-language pathologist confer about options for meeting Frenchy's hydration and nutrition needs. After reviewing the radiologist's report and viewing the videotape of the fluoroscopy, they decide that Frenchy should be given an NG tube. Because of the severity of her dysphagia and the global aphasia, therapies to improve her swallowing are contraindicated. They agree that after 2 or 3 weeks, another video swallow study will be done to see if the swallow has improved due to spontaneous recovery of sensory and motor functioning. Unfortunately, Frenchy also fails that test, and eventually a permanent gastric tube leading directly to her stomach is required.

Case Study 7.3 Dysphagia and Tracheotomy in a 32-Year-Old Man

ROBERT JOHNSON

Robert Johnson, an accountant with a chain of nursing homes, died of complications related to asthma. After his death, his parents set up a charitable fund in his name, and for several years, the university speech and hearing clinic, where he had received

Clinical Sidebar 7.3
Some patients with brain injury may be impulsive, risking choking and aspiration. They may place large amounts of food in their mouths, neglect to swallow, or attempt to talk during the swallow. Impulsive patients must be carefully monitored during meals. What procedure has helped save many choking victims? How is it performed?

dysarthria therapy, accepted donations in his name. Although Robert had taken a powerful medication, it was only marginally successful in controlling his asthma, particularly on dry, dusty days. Apparently, he had neglected to take it for several days prior to a nearly fatal asthma attack in the mistaken belief that he had improved and it was no longer needed. Robert also hated the side effects of the medication, especially the anxiety. On the day of the attack, he was working in his office, managing the accounts of hundreds of nursing home patients. An ambulance was summoned, and he was rushed to the nearest hospital in respiratory arrest. He suffered anoxia and his cerebellum took most of the damage, leaving him severely ataxic. Clinically, he was stuporous when transferred to the regional rehabilitation center. He was also on a respirator that pumped air into and out of his lungs through a tracheal tube.

Robert's levels of awareness and consciousness fluctuated. Sometimes he was alert and responsive; at other times, he was semicomatose. Ordinarily, a patient on a respirator would not be admitted to this rehabilitation center, but because of Robert's fluctuating levels of awareness and alertness, one goal was to wean him from the respirator. Another goal was to have him meet his hydration and nutrition needs orally. Before coming to the rehabilitation center, he was fed orally in the mistaken belief that with the cuff of the tracheotomy tube inflated, he could not aspirate. Robert had recurrent bouts of aspiration pneumonia in the acute care ward; the staff did not understand how he could aspirate with the trachea blocked by the inflated cuff.

After about 2 weeks in the rehabilitation center, Robert occasionally breathed on his own. He was fed a puree mixture by the nursing staff, and each time the cuff was inflated to the proper pressure. Nurses were perplexed at Robert's recurrent aspiration pneumonia. They had been taught that with the cuff inflated, there is no way food or liquid can penetrate the lower air passageways. Suspecting that remnant liquid and food particles were entering the lungs when the cuff was deflated, they took special care that no liquid or food remained when deflating the cuff. Yet, Robert continued to suffer from aspiration pneumonia. One nurse suspected that family members were providing him with food when the cuff was deflated.

To test for aspiration when the cuff was inflated, a dye was placed in the pureed food. Blue was chosen because it is not the color of naturally occurring body fluids. The cuff was then inflated to the required pressure, and the blue puree mix was placed in Robert's mouth. He managed to create a bolus and move it to the back of his throat. When it was in position, he swallowed. Then a nurse slid a small suction tube through the tracheal opening and gently down toward his lungs. Soon a bluish liquid could be seen going through the suction tube and into a container. Obviously, Robert had aspirated the puree even with the cuff inflated. Several tests were conducted using the blue dye while adjusting the pressure and placement of the tracheal cuff. Each time, dye penetrated Robert's lungs.

Robert returned to the acute wing of the hospital, where his trachea was examined endoscopically. The surgeon discovered that he had a fistula (hole) in the trachea that allowed pureed food and liquid into the air passageway. Apparently, the fistula was so large that no tracheal cuff placement or adjustment of pressure could stop the infiltration. The fistula was surgically repaired, and an NG tube was inserted while it healed. Thanks to the blue dye, the fistula had been discovered and Robert no longer suffered from recurrent aspiration pneumonia. Eventually, he was discharged from the rehabilitation center and received dysarthria therapy at the university speech and hearing clinic. Two years later, he suffered a fatal asthma attack.

Case Study 7.4   Dysphagia Associated with Partial Glossectomy in a 31-Year-Old Man

KEVIN

Kevin started smoking when he was 14 years old. He and his friend smoked two or three cigarettes while waiting for the school bus, and their parents never suspected that this was the reason for their leaving early for school. After graduation, Kevin took a job as a farm hand and began using chewing tobacco. Like baseball players of old, he chewed chopped tobacco and spit it onto the ground. He also liked to place a pinch of finely ground tobacco between his lower lip and gum. By the time Kevin was in his 30s, he was addicted to nicotine. Also an alcoholic, Kevin learned in Alcoholics Anonymous meetings that he had an *addictive personality.* It seemed he could not break pleasurable habits, and he used tobacco to excess. He loved the nicotine rush.

Kevin lived in a small mobile home provided by his employer. He spent days on the farm plowing fields, bailing hay, moving irrigation pipes, and harvesting wheat. Kevin was a hard worker and a good farm hand. He was also a chain smoker, usually lighting a new cigarette with an old one. In the evenings he chewed tobacco, and just before going to sleep, he put a pinch of the finely ground substance between his lower lip and gum. One day, he went to the dentist with a toothache and was told to see an ear, nose, and throat specialist. Kevin disliked going to doctors, but he followed instructions. The specialist performed several biopsies and told Kevin that he had oral cancer. Kevin was devastated; he had always denied the risk. He thought cancer was for older persons who had used tobacco for many years. That evening, he stopped using tobacco forever.

Clinical Sidebar 7.4
There is a strong scientifically demonstrated link between the use of tobacco products and oral-laryngeal cancers. Are the public announcements and the danger warnings on tobacco products reducing the number of users?

Kevin was admitted to the hospital and had several surgeries to remove the cancerous tumors. About one third of his tongue was surgically removed—a partial glossectomy. Part of his lower jaw and neck tissue were also excised to stop the deadly disease from spreading. Later, he underwent radiation therapy. The surgeries and therapy took about 6 months, and a major complication was difficulty swallowing. A tube was placed in his stomach, and five times a day Kevin poured a liquid into it with all the vitamins, minerals, and nutrients he needed. When the doctor believed the irradiated tissue and surgeries had healed and the soreness had subsided, he ordered a swallowing evaluation. It had been months since Kevin had taken food or liquid orally, and the only tasteful substance to enter his mouth was the lemon-flavored swabs he used to clean and moisten it.

The speech-language pathologist saw Kevin as an outpatient for the swallowing evaluation. It was held in the rehabilitation wing of the hospital, but because of the risk of choking and aspiration, it was done in a diagnostic room instead of an outpatient suite. The clinician told Kevin about the choking and aspiration risks, and wanted easy access to suction and emergency medical personnel if necessary.

The oral-facial evaluation showed the extent of the surgeries. The left side of Kevin's tongue had been almost completely removed. Much of his lower jaw bone had been destroyed, and there was scarring and indentation in his neck where muscles, glands, and tissue had been removed. Kevin's left lower molars and incisors were missing. Tongue mobility was limited for protrusion, retraction, lateralization, depression, and elevation. Intrinsic tongue muscles, particularly on the left side, were unable to adjust the shape of the tongue. Sensation was diminished throughout the left oral pharyngeal region.

Kevin's voice was unremarkable, with no voice quality change. He could not perform velopharyngeal closure to create the intraoral air pressure required to suck from a straw. However, by placing a straw on the right side of his mouth, he could suck water from a glass. Once the liquid was in his mouth, by keeping it to the right side, he was able to initiate a swallow. There was no seepage through his lips or into his nasal cavity. He could initiate a normal reflexive and purposeful swallow without choking or coughing. He also displayed successful oral containment, transportation, and swallowed ice chips, and could manage purees and finely chopped foods. Finely chopped meats required additional lubrication, which was provided by sauces and gravies.

Kevin underwent plastic surgery to reduce the scarring and deformation resulting from the cancer surgeries. Eventually, he returned to his job as a farm worker and learned to prepare meals to accommodate his oral limitations. Five years later, the time deemed necessary for a cure, the oral cancer had not returned.

Case Study 7.5   Isolated Dysphagia in a 47-Year-Old Man

JIM MANTEROLLA

The rehabilitation clerk gives you a message that a dysphagia evaluation has been ordered for a 47-year-old man in the intensive care unit. On arrival, you go to the nurses' station and ask for Jim Manterolla's chart.

The cover page has the usual information, such as the patient's full name, address, telephone and Social Security numbers, primary care physician, and payment sources. You take notes for the report you will write and are surprised at the admission diagnosis, which is simply one word: *dysphagia*. This seems unusual; dysphagia

Clinical Sidebar 7.5
According to the American Speech-Language-Hearing Association, in 1985, 35% of speech-language pathologists were involved in the diagnosis and treatment of dysphagia patients. By 1995, the percentage had increased to 52%. Today, most speech-language pathologists working in medical environments see patients with dysphagia. Some professionals believe that because dysphagia is not a communication disorder, it should not be part of the scope of practice of speech-language pathologists. What do you think?

generally occurs with traumatic brain injury, cerebrovascular accident, multiple sclerosis, amyotrophic lateral sclerosis, and other serious conditions.

You read the neurology and radiology reports to try to understand this patient's unusual medical predicament. They are not very helpful. The computed tomography scan shows no cerebral infarcts. This is not surprising; it takes several hours, and sometimes days, for a scan to show brain damage, and even then, small, isolated lesions may never be discovered. The neurology report suggests that the patient is free from illness. You skim the rest of the report and focus on "Impressions." The neurologist believes the dysphagia may be related to undetected damage of glossopharyngeal or vagus cranial nerves, and because of the rapid onset, the neurological damage is probably vascular in origin. As often happens when neurologists cannot pinpoint the site of the lesion, "possibly psychogenic in origin" is also stated.

You enter the patient's room and greet him. Mr. Manterolla is sitting on the side of the bed. He has a suction tube in his right hand and a towel folded on his lap. He returns your greeting articulately and with no indications of dysarthria. His voice quality is normal; in fact, his voice is strong and resonant. When he walks to the dresser to replace the towel, he moves normally. You ask several general questions and then ask him to explain what brought him to the intensive care unit.

He describes yesterday's medical emergency in vivid detail. He was working in his garden early in the morning to avoid the midday heat. He had just dug several holes and planted potatoes. At about 8:30, he noticed drool escaping from his mouth and could not seem to swallow. (At this point, he places the suction tube in his mouth, removes the accumulated liquid, and wipes his chin with the towel.) He tried several times to swallow and realized that something was wrong. He drove himself to the hospital, was promptly admitted, and has since been examined, probed, scanned, and evaluated. He spent a sleepless night suctioning and wiping liquid from his mouth. No one in the hospital would take the time to tell him what was wrong, and he was getting very frustrated.

You explain that a firm diagnosis has yet to be made. In addition, you describe your role in the diagnostic processes and explain that therapies exist to help him regain the ability to swallow. You also note that his isolated swallowing disorder is unusual.

The clinical/bedside screening reveals nothing remarkable about the oral intake and transportation stages of his swallow. Mr. Manterolla accepts ice chips and creates a bolus. There is good lip seal and mastication, and his dentition is unremarkable. There is no apparent pocketing in his cheeks. Tongue mobility and sensation are normal. He has no difficulty propelling the bolus along the palatal vault. Salivation is adequate to lubricate the bolus.

At the pharyngeal and esophageal-laryngeal levels there is no gag reflex, and possibly mild sensory deficits to the base of the tongue and posterior pharyngeal wall. However, no firm determination of sensation can be made due to the patient's inconsistent responses. He cannot initiate a swallow voluntarily or automatically, and there is no laryngeal elevation or apparent velopharyngeal closure. He has no concurrent motor speech disorders and no indications of apraxia of speech or the dysarthrias. His speech musculature shows no signs of flaccidity, spasticity, ataxia, hyperkinesis, or hypokinesis. At the conclusion of the clinical/bedside evaluation, the neurologist enters and beckons you to the nurses' station. Apparently, she wants to discuss Mr. Manterolla's case.

The neurologist is as perplexed about Mr. Manterolla's dysphagia as you are and explores several neurological possibilities. Lower motor neuron damage is ruled out because, as it is the final common pathway for motor movements, there would likely be accompanying flaccid paralysis or paresis. You confirm that there are no indications of flaccid dysarthria. Both of you agree that the site of the lesion must be above the glossopharyngeal-spinal accessory nucleus where the cell bodies are found. The neurologist believes that there may be a small lesion in the cranial nerve X-XI complex. Alternatively, the lesion may be higher in the motor control network involving motor speech programming: apraxic dysphagia. The neurologist suggests a possible psychological role in the dysphagia. Some neurological event may have precipitated it, but classically conditioned anxiety and associated negative emotions may be perpetuating it. You and the neurologist agree that the precise etiology of the dysphagia may never be discovered. You also agree that knowing the etiology, although helpful, is not necessary for treating it.

After another day of observation, Mr. Manterolla is discharged home. Over the next several weeks, you work with him on his swallowing disorder. You use a tongue blade to gently probe the back of his throat to elicit a gag reflex, massage the laryngeal muscles, and use behavior modification to increase laryngeal elevation during attempts to swallow. Gradually, spontaneous recovery occurs, the therapies produce results, and the necessary sensation and motor movements return to the posterior oral cavity. You use ice chips as swallowing stimuli, and one day, the patient voluntarily swallows them. Soon thereafter, Mr. Manterolla's swallowing reflex returns and he is able to eat normally. You discharge him, never knowing the true cause of his isolated dysphagia.

SUMMARY

Swallowing, defined broadly, includes the emotional, cognitive, sensory, and/or motor acts involved in transferring a substance from the mouth to the stomach. Dysphagia results in failure to maintain hydration and nutrition, and poses the risks of choking and aspiration. Only limited information can be obtained during a clinical/bedside screening; a video swallow study is often required. There are several commonsense changes in diet, and modification of chewing and swallowing behaviors, that can help patients regain the ability to meet their hydration and nutrition needs orally.

Study and Discussion Questions

1. Why have speech-language pathologists assumed a primary role in evaluation and treatment of dysphagia?

2. Define dysphagia.

3. Describe a normal swallow and explain how speech production is related to swallowing.

4. Describe the goals, procedures, and limitations of a clinical/bedside dysphagia evaluation.

5. What factors predict the severity of dysphagia?

6. Describe a video swallow study.

7. Describe nasogastric, gastric, and tracheal tubes and their use in patients with dysphagia.

8. What factors are involved in the diagnosis and treatment of dysphagia in geriatric and pediatric patients?

9. List and describe five dysphagia therapies.

10. Discuss false-positive and false-negative dysphagia test results.

Recommended Reading

Arvedson, J. C., & Brodsky, L. (2002). *Pediatric swallowing and feeding: Assessment and management* (2nd ed.). San Diego, CA: Singular.
    This book examines the unique aspects of pediatric dysphagia and feeding problems.

Cefalu, C. (1999). Appropriate dysphagia evaluation and management of the nursing home patient with dementia. *Annals of Long-Term Care, 7*(12), 447–451.
    This article addresses the diagnosis and treatment of swallowing disorders in patients with dementia.

Logemann, J. A. (1998). *Evaluation and treatment of swallowing disorders*. Austin, TX: Pro-Ed.
    This book addresses diagnosis and treatment of dysphagia in several populations.

Tanner, D. (2003). *The forensic aspects of communication sciences and disorders*. Tucson, AZ: Lawyers and Judges.
    Chapter 3 of this book examines dysphagia from a forensic and litigation perspective.

CHAPTER EIGHT

Traumatic Brain Injury

Not a sentence or a word is independent of the circumstances under which it is uttered.

Alfred North Whitehead

Chapter Preview: This chapter describes communication disorders resulting from traumatic brain injuries. Open and closed head injuries are considered, as well as the communication disorders associated with them. There is also a discussion of orientation, memory, and behavior problems typically see in patients with traumatic brain injury. Case studies include a 17-year-old girl with an open head injury following a suicide attempt, and two adults and a child who suffered brain damage because of motor vehicle accidents. There is an account of response delay and long-term effects of traumatic brain injury, as well as a case involving a motorcycle accident victim in an eye-open vegetative state.

OVERVIEW OF TRAUMATIC BRAIN INJURY AND COMMUNICATION DISORDERS

In the United States, there are about 500,000 **traumatic brain injury** hospitalizations each year (Ylvisaker, Szekeres, & Feeney, 2001). Although some persons die of these injuries, many survive. The survival rate has increased because of medical and technological advances. Today, there are ambulance, helicopter, and airplane rapid transportation services from accident sites to trauma centers where doctors and nurses can relieve the dangerous pressure within the skull that often develops with serious traumatic brain injury. According to Ghajar (2002), the improved outcome for patients with severe traumatic brain injury is attributed to reducing this pressure and increasing blood flow to the brain.

Head-Injured Persons

Several studies have focused on the types of persons who suffer traumatic brain injuries. All studies show that men, particularly young ones, are at least twice as likely as women to be involved. Hickey (1997) reports that about 50% of all head injuries are caused by motor vehicle accidents, followed by falls (21%) and assaults and violence (12%). "In the very young and in the elderly, the primary cause of injury is falls, whereas ABI [accidental brain injury] in young adults is more likely to be caused by accidents and assaults"

(Petit, 2001, p. 70). Drug and alcohol use, as well as risky jobs and recreational activities, are also positively correlated with traumatic brain injuries. Interestingly, persons who are admitted to a hospital for a traumatic brain injury are likely to have been previously hospitalized for a similar injury. The following is a profile of the typical head-injured person:

> A young single male with poor education and academic skills, working in a job where the risk of accidental injury is great, earning below average income, who engages in risk-taking behaviors while using alcohol or recreational drugs, and who has previously been admitted to a hospital for a traumatic head and neck injury. (Tanner, 2003b, p. 118)

There are two types of head injuries: open and closed. An **open head injury** occurs when an object—a **projectile** or **missile**—penetrates the skull and brain. A common projectile in an open head injury is a bullet fired from a gun. Others include shrapnel from a bomb explosion and bolts or tools falling from high places in industrial accidents. Projectiles and missiles damage the brain when they impact and enter it.

A **closed head injury** occurs when an object impacts but does not penetrate the skull and brain. These injuries are often caused by blunt blows. The force of the blow causes the brain to **accelerate** and **decelerate**. Often rotational acceleration of the brain results in shearing of **axons** (Gillis & Pierce, 1996), the parts of the brain that carry nerve impulses away from cell bodies. The brain is suddenly accelerated by the force of the blow and it rotates, tearing and shearing the axons within.

Open and closed head injuries can cause **focalized** and **diffuse** brain injury. Focalized injury affects one identifiable area of the brain. Diffuse injury involves more than one site. In some types of head injury, brain damage is primarily limited to one area. Many high-impact head injuries produce **coup** and **contra-coup** effects. The coup effect occurs at the site of the initial impact. The contra-coup effect is on the opposite side of the brain because of one of the laws of physics: for every action, there is an equal and opposite reaction. This damage occurs because of the recoil of the brain inside the skull. "If the head is not immobilized when struck, the majority of the injury may be to the brain on the opposite side of the head from impact—a 'contra-coup' injury" (Fuller & Goodman, 2001, p. 281).

Neurogenic Communication Disorders and Traumatic Brain Injury

To a limited extent, the site or sites of the brain damage determines the patient's communication disorder. If the primary speech and language centers of the brain are damaged, there may be one or more neurogenic communication disorder. When the damage is limited to these areas, patients present with symptoms of classic aphasia, apraxia of speech, and dysarthria typically seen in stroke patients. Aphasia caused by focalized cerebral lesions occurs in approximately 6% of cases of traumatic brain injury (Petit, 2001). In some cases, although patients suffer brain damage, the major speech and language centers are spared. They do not have the classic symptoms of aphasia, apraxia of speech, and the dysarthrias. These patients may have **language of confusion**. The brain damage causes reduced or impaired **consciousness**, and their speech and language reflect the confusion.

In many patients with traumatic brain injuries, the neurogenic communication disorders are **complicated** by reduced or impaired consciousness. They have the slurred, indistinct speech of dysarthria, the motor speech programming problems of apraxia of speech, and the aphasic word finding and naming deficits occurring in the cloud of confusion. The confusion results in unusual and sometimes bizarre symptoms. They make random naming errors or produce unintelligible utterances and sometimes act as if the listeners should understand their "perfectly normal" speech. Their communication is not only disrupted by the damaged speech and language centers of the brain but also affected by the global confusion.

Coma

Not all patients who have serious traumatic brain injuries become comatose, and **coma** can happen in other neurological events such as stroke. However, many patients who suffer traumatic brain injuries become comatose, and their awareness of self and the environment is reduced or impaired to varying degrees—**stupor**, **delirium**, and **clouding of consciousness**. The patient in stupor requires continued stimulation to be aroused. Delirium is associated with confusion, and the patient is agitated. In clouding of consciousness, the mildest level of reduced awareness, the patient is mildly confused and may at times appear normal.

The Glasgow Coma Scale (Teasdale & Jennett, 1974) is a test widely used to measure the degree of coma. It assesses the patient's eye-opening, motor response, and speech; scores range from 3 to 15. The Rancho Los Amigos Scale (Malkmus, Booth, & Kodimer, 1980), another widely used test of cognitive and behavioral functioning, can be used to help family members understand the process of recovery (Mackay, Chapman, & Morgan, 1997). This test has eight cognitive levels (e.g., "no response," "confused, agitated," "automatic, appropriate") and a description of behaviors; it also gives suggestions for patient management.

Traumatic Brain Injury, Disorientation, and Amnesia

Amnesia and **disorientation** go hand-in-hand in many patients with traumatic brain injuries. Amnesia is memory loss, and the time of the accident is the dividing line for detecting the loss of memories for past events (**retrograde** amnesia) and the inability to acquire new memories (**anterograde** amnesia). Retrograde amnesia can be as brief as a few hours or as long as several years and even decades. It is related to disorientation because memory of past events is necessary for orientation to time, people, places, and situations.

Many patients with serious traumatic brain injuries are disoriented at some time during the recovery period. Such patients have lost their bearing. The most common type of disorientation involves **time**. Disorientation to time includes the time of events and the passage of time. For patients completely disoriented to time, these concepts are lost. These patients may also have forgotten one or several of the **persons** in their lives. Disorientation to relationship can include family and friends. Patients may even lose their sense of identity. Confusion about what happened and the cause of the hospitalization is called disorientation to **situation** or **predicament**. Disorientation to **place** is not knowing one or more physical locations. Usually, patients are disoriented about several aspects of reality, but some are only disoriented about one. A patient disoriented to one aspect of reality is said to be disoriented **times one**, disorientation to two aspects of reality is called disorientation **times two**, and so forth. A person who is completely disoriented is said to be disoriented **times four**: time, place, person, and situation (predicament).

Retrograde and Anterograde Amnesia

As noted above, retrograde amnesia is loss of memory before the traumatic brain injury. This type of amnesia can be caused by organic and psychological factors. Many patients cannot remember the event that caused the brain damage.

The organic factors causing amnesia about the causative incident involve changes in brain chemistry. An important brain structure for memory is the hippocampus. Injury of this structure, and of other parts of the brain, can produce a change in brain chemistry leading to loss of memory of the incident. The psychological factor associated with posttraumatic amnesia for the incident is **repression** (Tanner, 2003a), a protective defense mechanism used to block memories of distressing or threatening events. Repression occurs **subconsciously**, outside of the person's awareness. Organic changes in the brain and repression account for cases of amnesia for the incident that caused the traumatic brain injury.

Anterograde amnesia affects the acquisition of new memories. It can be minimal, involving only memory for events immediately after the accident, or it can be extensive, destroying the ability to learn new information. Although both retrograde and anterograde amnesia can be significant in the patient's recovery, the ability to lay down new memories is essential to rehabilitation. It is necessary to profit from experience, and thus benefit from teaching, training, and counseling.

Both **short-term** and **long-term** processes are involved in learning and acquiring new memories. Short-term memory includes attending to and remembering information while rehearsing it. Remembering a telephone number is a good example. The average person can remember seven numbers, with a range from five to nine. In the United States, local telephone numbers are seven digits in length. After the number is looked up in the telephone book, it can be remembered as long as the person rehearses it, either aloud or in the mind. However, if the person is interrupted during the rehearsal, the number is lost and must be looked up again. In long-term memory, the number is remembered even when it is not rehearsed. Numbers are associated with other information in the person's mind. With long-term storage, new information is available for purposeful or incidental recall.

Metacognition, Mental Executive Functioning, and Traumatic Brain Injury

Executive functioning is the mental ability to execute, regulate, plan, and monitor behaviors and actions. The idea comes from business, where the top executive of a corporation is responsible for running it and monitoring its affairs. Executive functioning is part of **metacognition**: thinking about thinking. Metacognition is the monitoring of cognitive processes (Gillis, 1996). It encompasses knowing how and when to attend to information and when and what to remember. Metacognition is knowing when problems exist and strategies for solving them. It is a more encompassing concept than executive functioning and accounts for the behavior problems seen in persons with traumatic brain injury.

Traumatic Brain Injury and Behavioral Problems

The behavior of many patients changes during recovery from traumatic brain injury. Early on, they may be unresponsive; gradually, they become more responsive to persons and things. They may also become withdrawn and distant or agitated and aggressive. Many of these changes in behavior are seen as temporary and necessary stages in recovery.

Some patients with traumatic brain injury become **socially disinhibited**, no longer appreciating and instead violating societal norms. Many of these violations involve sexual behaviors. Sometimes patients lose their modesty and enter public places partially or completely unclothed. Sexual drives may be misdirected and inappropriate. Patients may become **hypersexual** and appear to lose sexual regulatory functions. Some of them proposition medical staff and visitors and make sexually suggestive remarks to strangers.

Patients with traumatic brain injury may also be aggressive and even violent. In the blur of confusion, they may strike out and injure staff, family, and friends. Some of them are verbally aggressive and dismissive of others. Patients may be excessively territorial, not allowing others to enter their room or sit with them at the dinner table.

Whereas some patients are agitated and aggressive, others are indifferent and seem emotionally distant from family and friends, a condition called **flat affect**. *Affect* refers to the emotions associated with a thought and how they are manifested. Patients with flat affect appear unconcerned about others, even friends and relatives, and thoughts about their predicament are not accompanied by the expected emotions. They do not display the emotions experienced by normal persons under similar circumstances. Family and friends often report that the patient's unusual reactions to persons, things, and situations are chronic personality changes following traumatic brain injury.

In **response delay**, another common behavior change seen in patients with traumatic brain injury, the patient takes excessive time to perform certain tasks. This is particularly apparent in taking turns during conversations. In turn-taking, timing is important. If one person talks longer than is acceptable, the other may interrupt. Patients with response delay may take much longer than usual to answer a question or make a remark. They appear to be processing information very slowly or to have tense speech muscles that cannot be moved. Also, some patients, particularly those with damage to the frontal lobes, lack initiative. This reduced spontaneity, when combined with spastic speech muscles, sometimes produces extremely long response delays.

Posttraumatic Psychosis

Posttraumatic psychosis is a generic label for psychotic illness in a person who has suffered a traumatic brain injury; it may affect as many as 50% of these patients (Smeltzer, Nasrallah, & Miller, 1994). Patients with posttraumatic psychosis have problems with **reality testing** and often develop **hallucinations** and **delusions**. Hallucinations are false or

Table 8.1 Cognitive, Behavioral, and Communication Disorders in Traumatic Brain Injury

Function	Disorder	Description
Awareness	Coma, stupor, delirium, clouding of consciousness	Absent or reduced awareness of self and environment
Reality testing	Posttraumatic psychosis	Break with one or more aspects of reality: hallucinations and delusions
Memory	Retrograde and anterograde amnesia	Memory loss of events before or after the traumatic brain injury; problems learning
Orientation	Disorientation to time, place, person, or situation (predicament)	Confusion about time of events or the passage of time, persons (including self), place, and the reason for hospitalization
Communication	Neurogenic communication disorders; language of confusion	Motor speech disorders and language deficits; communication acts indicative of impairments of awareness, memory, orientation, and reality testing

distorted interpretations of information coming from the senses. Delusions are false beliefs that are rigidly held even in the face of proof to the contrary. The diagnosis of posttraumatic psychosis is difficult when the patient suffers from communication disorders such as aphasia. The patient may appear to be experiencing delusions and hallucinations when, in fact, he or she is simply reporting real events with paraphasias. Table 8.1 lists the prominent cognitive, behavioral, and communication disorders of traumatic brain injury.

Pediatric Traumatic Brain Injury

Children with traumatic brain injury often have a better prognosis for rehabilitation than adults, but they also have unique challenges. Because a young person's brain is more pliant than that of an adult, when a particular area is damaged, other areas of the brain may more readily take over the lost functions. Children with traumatic brain injury may also compensate more easily for impaired function by learning to work around deficiencies and using existing strengths. On the negative side, children may be more vulnerable than older people in certain critical areas of functioning (Ylvisaker, 1998). Unlike many adults with traumatic brain injuries, rehabilitation for the child involves returning to school and a lengthy period of formal learning. Teaching and learning strategies for the child must be adjusted to accommodate the cognitive, behavioral, and emotional changes resulting from the injury. And of course, children are in a period of rapid mental, physical, and emotional growth, and have different perspectives and needs. For example, family support and peer acceptance are more important for children than for most adults.

Treatment of Communication Disorders in Traumatic Brain Injury

It has been said that rehabilitation for the patient with traumatic brain injury begins at the accident site. In rehabilitation, an early start ensures that all that can be done will be done. Unfortunately, some patients with severe traumatic brain injuries do not survive, and others may never recover from deep comas. Remarkably, some patients make a complete recovery. Many patients improve considerably and go on to enjoy functional and independent lives.

For patients with significantly reduced consciousness, the goal of rehabilitation is to improve general awareness, orientation, responsiveness, and the ability to learn. In some patients, the use of psychostimulants may improve attention and reduce distractibility, disorganization, hyperactivity, impulsiveness, and emotional lability (Petit, 2001).

Coma stimulation is an experimental therapy that provides the patient with multisensory stimulation to improve responsiveness. There are several coma stimulation techniques. Some involve reading to the patient, massaging the body, placing different odors and fragrances under the nose, and so forth. The goal is to stimulate the patient to improve arousal, awareness, alertness, and the general ability to benefit from rehabilitation. Some patients, particularly those with higher levels of awareness, may respond to this type of stimulation. Certain clinicians believe that coma stimulation, even for patients in deep comas, increases the likelihood that the patient will make greater gains in rehabilitation after recovering from the coma. Unfortunately, this therapy has not been carefully researched and proven to benefit comatose patients. It provides the patient's family and friends with activities to reduce their sense of helplessness, such as reading to the patient, talking about current events, and providing nurturing statements. However, it is important for them to understand that for most patients in a deep coma, little can be done to improve awareness. Current medications, technology, and therapeutic procedures do not significantly improve consciousness in most of these patients. Desperate families may grasp at any technique to help their loved ones (Gillis, 1996), but false hope and unrealistic expectations should not be created.

Rehabilitation of patients with traumatic brain injuries involves the team approach. The primary team members usually include attending physicians, physiatrists (specialists in physical medicine and rehabilitation), nurses, dietitians, neuropsychologists, social workers, speech-language pathologists, and occupational and physical therapists. Other specialists, such as psychiatrists, pediatric neurologists, gerontologists, music therapists, and rehabilitation counselors, may be called on to join the team, depending on case-specific requirements. According to Mackay et al. (1997), patients with traumatic brain injury should also be seen by an audiologist to establish the likelihood of damage to auditory structures.

With regard to communication, there are two primary treatment foci for patients with traumatic brain injuries. First, the patient's mental executive functioning and metacognition abilities are addressed to improve his or her behavior, memory, orientation, and learning. **Reality orientation** is a procedure used in many rehabilitation facilities to achieve these goals. In it, all team members tell the patient the time and date, the reason for seeing the patient, and other pertinent information. The goal is to provide ongoing, consistent information to help the patient reorient to the new circumstances. The team, including the patient's family, also works on behavioral objectives, which include rewarding appropriate behaviors and discouraging inappropriate ones. Consistency is important in the rehabilitation of traumatic brain-injured persons, and the team meets regularly to plan goals and objectives, provide treatments, and monitor outcomes.

The second focal area is the specific neurogenic communication disorder. Patients with dysarthria are given the appropriate neuromuscular therapies to improve respiration, phonation, articulation, resonance, and prosody. Apraxia of speech therapy improves motor speech conceptualization, programming, and planning. Aphasia therapies address expressive and receptive language deficits in all affected modalities. The therapies for neurogenic communication disorders in patients who also have metacognition and mental executive deficits require special modifications for their memory, orientation, and behavioral problems.

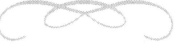

Case Studies in Traumatic Brain Injury and Communication Disorders

Case Study 8.1 Open Head Injury After a Suicide Attempt

CANDACE

For Candace, a high school junior, her first love was like a wild roller-coaster ride filled with the euphoria of young, passionate love and, in the end, the desperation and pain of rejection. Briefly, it was the best and the worst of times. Tragically, Candace's first love ended in a suicide attempt and a severe traumatic brain injury due to a self-inflicted gunshot wound to the head. A cheating boyfriend, drunkenness, and the anguish of rejection forever changed her life and the lives of her family and friends.

Candace was born on a large cattle ranch in the picturesque Teton Mountain Range of Wyoming. An only child, she had doting parents and grew to love horses and the wide-open spaces. Ranch work is hard, but Candace gladly accepted the responsibilities of tending to suckling calves and bum lambs. She had little time for school activities, given her after-school chores and the need to care for abandoned animals. An honor student, Candace was popular with her schoolmates, and had typical "puppy loves" and infatuations. Then, in her junior year, one of the "bad boys" at school stole her heart. Her parents forbade the relationship, which seemed to make it all the more special. For several months, their love grew and blossomed.

One spring evening when her parents were away from home, Candace had a party. Several couples and singles from her school came, and her boyfriend brought beer. A wild time was had by all. Late that night a gunshot rang out. A panicked and distraught Candace had put her father's pistol to her head and pulled the trigger. The pain of seeing her boyfriend in the embrace of another girl was more than she could handle, and in a drunken blur she tried, and failed, to take her life.

The powerful pistol shot penetrated Candace's head and tore through the frontal lobes of her brain. She was immediately rushed to the only hospital in the county, and physicians and nurses worked for hours to save her life. Candace survived but was forever changed by the damage the gunshot caused to her brain.

For weeks, she lay in a coma. Doctors, nurses, and aides attended to her, changed the bandages on her head, and carefully fed her needed fluid and protein through a tube inserted though her nose that led to her stomach. Candace remained unresponsive to all external and internal stimulation. Fortunately, she was spared the psychological pain of the tragedy endured by those closest to her.

Her parents and friends visited her regularly and tried desperately to awaken her from the deep coma. Over the next few months, Candace was transferred to the hospital's acute care ward and finally to the rehabilitation unit for coma stimulation. She lay silently in bed, only occasionally opening her eyes, detached from those who tried to reach her. When she did open her eyes, she did not look at the sources of sounds, visually track persons and things, or even startle at loud noises. Curiously, she made baby-like sucking actions with her lips when her mother stroked her arm and tried to comfort her.

Clinical Sidebar 8.1
A patient in a coma may appear to be asleep, but the two states are fundamentally different. Also, studies have shown that a patient in a coma may go through the same stages of sleep seen in normal persons. Do you know anyone who has emerged from a coma after several years? Did he or she recall events that happened during the coma?

Coma stimulation involved all of the senses. The goal was to arouse Candace and create the general ability to attend to persons and new information. Candace's parents and the doctors, nurses, and therapists hoped it would reduce her coma and improve her rehabilitation potential. Different odors and fragrances were placed under her nose, contrasting temperatures and textures were applied to her skin, and different types of sounds penetrated her ears. She was read newspapers and magazines and given full-body massages. Even her playful puppy was brought from the ranch and carefully placed on her lap. But it was to no avail. Although the stimulation did provide her parents and friends with activities to reduce their sense of helplessness, nothing could arouse Candace from her coma.

After many painful months, Candace's parents and friends accepted the new reality: there were no medications, doctors, or therapies capable of bringing Candace out of her stupor. Her head wound healed, although an indentation remained in her forehead. Several months later, Candace was transferred to a nursing home, where she spent her remaining days oblivious to family, friends, and the life and love she once knew.

Case Study 8.2   Closed Head Injury and Amnesia After a Motor Vehicle Accident

ANNA WANAMAKER

The Wanamakers were beginning life anew. Jerry and Anna quit their high-paying jobs, packed up their children and belongings, and began the long journey from California to Iowa. Five years ago, they had met at work when Anna had taken the prize job as the Southern California district sales representative for a large high-tech computer company. Both had previously divorced, and finding each other in the chaos of the single world was a blessing. Their casual friendship at work slowly blossomed into mature love. Their wedding had been a traditional one, with standard vows, children as ring bearers and ushers, rice, and a brief, practical honeymoon. The Wanamakers took pride in their practicality, but they also had dreams. The move from California to Iowa was to be a dream come true. Tragically, it turned into a nightmare outside of Flagstaff, Arizona. A snow-packed interstate highway, poor visibility, and huge out-of-control, tractor-trailer trucks prematurely ended their dream.

Realtors are quick to note that when purchasing real estate, location largely determines its value. This dictum made Jerry and Anna's dream a possibility. During a summer visit to his Iowa farm family, Jerry noticed that the neighbor's farm was for sale—160 prime acres of land, with all of its machinery, outbuildings, and a large four-bedroom home. Amazingly, Jerry and Anna found that they could purchase it with the sale of their fixer-upper California home. Property values had soared in California and sunk in Iowa. For Jerry and Anna, location had made their dream a reality.

The night before their cross-country journey, their friends from work threw a big going-away party. Punch was drunk, tears were shed, and parting gifts were given. The party ended at 9:00 p.m., for the Wanamakers needed an early start. At sunrise the next morning, with their two children in the backseat of the sedan, seat belts securely fastened, they bid farewell to California and began their dream. California traffic was sparse during the early morning, and though there was a light rain, they made good time. Five hours later, they crossed into Arizona. Later, in Kingman, Arizona, they lunched and gassed the car. Two hours later, the Wanamakers began the climb into the mountains and pine trees of the state. Gradually, the rain turned to snow. Soon the snow was heavy, visibility was limited, and the initial slush had turned to ice. They could barely read the sign welcoming them to Flagstaff at an elevation of 7,000 feet. Then, in the distance, Anna thought she saw several buildings on the freeway. Panic engulfed her and Jerry as they realized they were seeing huge tractor-trailer trucks, crashed and crumpled ahead of them. The brakes of the car did little good, and they crashed into a jackknifed truck loaded with produce. The trucks behind them, traveling too fast and recklessly, slammed into their car and toppled onto others, and a deadly chain reaction ensued. That snowy, winter day, six people lost their lives and Anna lost her memory and speech.

Jerry and the children walked away from the crash without a scratch, but the jaws-of-life was necessary to separate Anna from the car. She was then placed in an ambulance and transported to the nearest hospital. During the accident, the roof of the car had collapsed on her head, causing a serious closed head injury. At the hospital her head was cleaned and shaved, and a neurosurgeon suctioned the blood clot from inside her brain and stopped the bleeding. The dangerous pressure within the brain was relieved and the blood supply restored. Jerry and the children spent an anxious evening in the lonely surgery waiting room, and early the next morning, the doctors announced that Anna would survive.

Clinical Sidebar 8.2
The meninges are three membranes covering the brain and spinal cord: the dura mater, arachnoid mata, and pia mata. Removal of a blood clot below the dura mata meninx is called *evacuation of a subdural hematoma.* What is meningitis, and what causes it?

After 3 weeks of hospitalization and nearly 2 months in a rehabilitation facility, Anna, with Jerry and the children, resumed their lives. At the farm, Anna used the newly constructed wheelchair ramp to enter the house, of which she had absolutely no recollection. She could barely talk to her new neighbors, and always had a slur requiring many repetitions. Anna had no memory of the accident. In fact, she had no memory of that dreadful day, the going-away party the night before, or her job at the computer company. Even her memories of Jerry and the children were checkered. But over the years, some memories gradually returned or were relearned from recollections told to her. Several years later, the insurance companies of the two trucking firms paid for her mental, physical, and communication disabilities—an empty attempt to compensate for the memories and dreams destroyed on that snowy winter day in Flagstaff, Arizona.

Case Study **8.3** Closed Head Injury After an Industrial Accident

BEN LAWTON

Standing straight and alert and using his index finger, Ben pulls the constricting shirt collar away from his windpipe. He looks down the church aisle of seated friends and relatives and sees Julie, his beautiful bride. At the sight of her, his anxiety slips away; he remembers the reason for this ceremony. Ben and Julie are beginning their lives together. Death, and a traumatic brain injury, nearly prevented this union. Three years ago, Ben had fallen from a ladder when almost lethal bolts of electricity shot through his body, causing him to slam to the floor of the nearly completed College Plaza Shopping Center. He had narrowly escaped death, but symptoms of his head trauma lingered.

As a journeyman electrician, Ben understood and respected electricity. The afternoon of his injury was one of routine final checks of the mall's lighting. When switches and circuit breakers were thrown, the lights burned brightly except those designed to illuminate the way to the men's rest room. Ben agreed to investigate, and a coworker offered to cut the power. After spreading the 10-foot metal stepladder, Ben, with electrician tools dangling from his belt, climbed to the highest perch of the ladder and began to test the wires. The thick industrial wires were difficult to pull and straighten. As he struggled with one of them, a bolt of electricity, grounded by the ladder, shot through him. Ben's body spasmed and he toppled off the ladder, falling to the floor. He laid there bleeding from a surface cut on the left side of his head, with entrance and exit electrical burns on his hand and leg. At least that's what people told him. Ben couldn't remember the fall or even the day it happened.

As Julie continues to walk down the aisle, Ben thinks about how fortunate he is to be wed this day. Though he has survived the electrical shock, the fall from the ladder, and the traumatic brain injury, word-finding problems persist. Worst of all, the accident has shaken his confidence. Ben knows the inescapable reality: he has suffered irreversible brain damage.

The weeks that followed the accident were a blur. Ben had spotty memories of therapists, nurses, and doctors. He remembered visits from his parents, friends, and

Clinical Sidebar 8.3
When helping patients to relearn words and their meanings, it is clinically desirable to emphasize words that are relevant and important to the patient. The goal is to start with words such as the names of body parts, clothing, work tools, family members, and so forth, and gradually expand to less egocentric words. Why do clinicians concentrate on words that are personally relevant to the patient? Why not work on infrequently used and unusual words?

fiancé, but the timing of their visits was confused. Ben's first vivid memory of his communication disorder, and the long rehabilitation road before him, occurred when his therapist brought his electrician's toolbox to the therapy suite. She opened it and asked Ben to name the tools. Ben had lived with the red toolbox, with its pliers, snips, tapes, screwdrivers, vice grips, meters, and wire caps, for nearly a decade. However, when he was asked to name them, no words came to mind. But the real anxiety occurred when he supplied words that were clearly wrong. Ben had a nagging suspicion that they were incorrect, but no matter how hard he tried, he could not recall the correct ones. During months of aphasia therapy, Ben gradually relearned the language of his previous vocation.

Julie takes her place at Ben's side. With both of them standing before the minister, Ben recalls recent instances when his word-finding problems had made him the butt of jokes. He fears he may again say something ridiculous, embarrassing his bride, ruining the ceremony, and preventing the wedding. He carefully rehearses the two important words: "I do."

Ben admits to himself that the errors at which his friends laughed were indeed funny and seemed to happen when he was excited. Recently, when his golden retriever, Fluffer, had five puppies, Ben announced their birth: "Fluffer had fluffies." Last week, when running to catch an elevator, he had asked the rider to "Hold the alligator," again bringing laughter to his friends and a puzzled look to the rider's face. And when he announced that Julie was considering being a stay-at-home "wifehouse," at first he couldn't understand his best friend's laughter. Only when the correct word order was supplied did Ben see the error of his speech. Anxiety builds as Ben continues to rehearse the words soon to be required of him: "I do."

Finally, Julie and Ben face the minister. His best man, who had found so much humor in his misnaming of an elevator, provides the ring. Julie takes her vows and then the minister looks at Ben. The time has come, and Ben hopes he will avoid a stupid verbal mistake. He then utters the two important words, "I do," with accuracy and precision, and the ceremony ends. Ben and Julie are now wed, and once again, Ben has won his ongoing battle over the traumatic brain injury he suffered 3 years ago.

Case Study **8.4** Closed Head Injury After a Motor Vehicle Accident

LANE RENFROE

High school is a time of testing boundaries and learning limits, but sometimes there are dire consequences. For Lane Renfroe, a night of car racing ended in the death of his best friend and his own confinement to a nursing home.

Lane, a high school senior, put every penny he earned into his restored 1967 Camaro Super Sport. What a great car! It was a quarter-mile racing marvel, a machine few drivers dared challenge. Restoring it was Lane's calling in life, and everyone in his high school admired his skill and bravery during the late-night races on the outskirts of the city. The Camaro was Lane's identity. Tragically, the crash that cost him his future, and his best friend's life, was caused by a blown front tire. The car flipped end-over-end, throwing Lane and his friend to the pavement. Death and permanent disability were the only spoils of that late-night race.

A person in his early 20s is out of place in a nursing home, but after months of rehabilitation, the doctors had decided that Lane had a poor prognosis for independent living. The nursing home was the only alternative. The car crash had damaged several surface areas of Lane's brain and compressed his brain stem. It had taken months for him to become even partially responsive to his inner needs and the environment. At first, he was agitated and needed to be restrained by a vest with straps securing him to his bed. Once he had broken loose from the restraints and tumbled to the floor, causing bruises and a bloody nose. Periodically, the restraints were removed, and Lane sat up in a specially designed chair and participated in therapies. He was slowly improving, although he had difficulty remembering the names of people and things. He had typical aphasic word-finding errors (paraphasias) in which he supplied a word that was associated with the correct one. For example, a *pen* was called a *pencil,* a *knife* was a *spoon,* and *socks* were *shoes.* Then one day, a psychologist erroneously diagnosed Lane with posttraumatic psychosis, believing that he suffered from delusions. Lane apparently believed that the medical staff, in a gesture of kindness, had placed him in a car and transported him to the nearby fire station.

During the psychological evaluation, Lane, using slurred but intelligible speech, reported that during the previous evening, people took him from his room, put him in a car, and drove him to the fire station. Several times he told this story, each time with an excited look on his face. The psychologist suspected that the story was false because of Lane's medical status and physical limitations. The nurses confirmed her suspicion. In fact, they had watched him carefully the previous evening.

In reality, Lane was not delusional; he had simply reported an actual event using aphasic paraphasias. In this nursing home, some patients were allowed to sit at the nurses' station as a reward for good behavior. For many patients, this was a prize worth the energy of participating fully in therapies, eating well, and keeping their rooms clean. It so happened that the place of honor was below a large glass-enclosed fire hose and extinguisher. Indeed, the previous evening, a nurse and an orderly had entered Lane's room, placed him in a wheelchair, and transported him there. Lane simply reported this event using aphasic paraphasias: *car* for *wheelchair, drove* for *wheeled,* and *fire station* for *fire hose.* After the misunderstanding was clarified, the diagnosis of posttraumatic psychosis was removed from Lane's chart. For Lane Renfroe, the high-speed car accident had brought many terrible consequences, but a delusional trip to a fire station was not one of them.

Clinical Sidebar 8.4
In verbal paraphasia, the patient utters a word that is semantically related to the correct one—an association error. A literal paraphasia occurs when the patient produces a word that is phonemically similar to the correct one—an approximation error. What are random naming errors, and is any naming error truly random? What might prompt such an error?

Case Study **8.5** Closed Head Injury from an Equestrian Accident

JOHNNY HENRON

Horses had always been a big part of Johnny Henron's life; he got his first horse when he was just 6 years old. He named her Flicka, and she became his best friend. Johnny trained and "broke" the colt for saddle, and she became a prized cattle horse. For Johnny and his parents, horses were not a hobby or pastime; they were an integral part of their Arizona ranch. Horses were necessary to herd cattle, and no stray could surpass Johnny and Flicka's teamwork.

In high school, Johnny married his sweetheart, Juanita, and, after graduation, landed a job as a cowboy on a large cattle ranch. Johnny and Juanita had three daughters and worked hard to save money to purchase their own ranch. One responsibility of a cowboy is "breaking" wild horses into obedience, and it was an Appaloosa stallion that cost Johnny his family.

Johnny was smart, and smart cowboys do not simply throw a bridle and saddle on a bronco, step into the stirrups, and hang on to the saddle horn for dear life. Johnny had learned from Flicka that the best way to break a horse is to be firm but gentle and gradually gain the horse's trust. So, he penned the Appaloosa stallion, fed him hay and grain, and offered him apples and sugar cubes as treats. A few days later, he calmly approached the horse and slipped on the bridle. Later, the horse allowed Johnny to put on a blanket and saddle and to lead him around the small corral. The horse balked at the saddle and bucked to remove it from his back. Johnny performed the same ritual for several days, and early one Sunday morning he slipped into the saddle. At first, the horse bucked a little to remove him, but gradually he began to tolerate the new weight of the saddle and rider. Over the next few weeks, horse and rider became a team. The day of the accident, when the reins fell to the ground, the horse obediently stayed by the fallen rider until help arrived.

One crisp autumn evening, while returning to the corral, Johnny decided to give the stallion its rein. The horse began a slow gallop and sped to an open, unrestrained dead run. Then, unexpectedly, a diamondback rattlesnake hidden in the sagebrush struck at the horse's front feet. The Appaloosa abruptly stopped, reared onto his hind legs, and threw Johnny to the ground. During the fall, his forward-moving head struck the horse's rearing head with enormous force, knocking him unconscious. The impact ruptured blood vessels in the frontal lobes of Johnny's brain and fractured his nose and jaw. He laid in a clump of sagebrush for several hours until he was discovered, placed in a pickup truck, and taken to a nearby dirt road, where an ambulance rushed him to a hospital.

Everyone knew Johnny and Juanita's marriage was in trouble. Perhaps it was the strain of their jobs, ever-present money problems, lack of communication, or a combination of stressors. Before the accident they had separated twice, and were in weekly counseling in a desperate attempt to save their marriage. Six months after the accident, Juanita filed for divorce and custody of their daughters. The accident and Johnny's condition had ended all hope of saving their marriage. Juanita had been offered a job by her uncle in Texas, and it was time for her and the children to move on.

The diagnosis on Johnny's chart was "frontal lobe syndrome secondary to closed head injury." Patients with frontal lobe syndrome have problems with metacognition and mental executive functioning, as well as perseveration, shallow or labile emotions, and a tendency toward concrete thinking. Johnny had all of these symptoms and a significant response delay, which usually occurs with major frontal lobe brain damage. His response delay was mournfully apparent when Juanita and his daughters bid him farewell on the day they began their journey to Texas.

Nurses, aides, orderlies, doctors, therapists, and some of the other patients know about the impending farewell visit from Juanita and the children. The halls were unusually quiet and somber as visiting hours approached. Johnny lay in his bed, staring at a television mounted in the corner of the room, apparently watching a talk show. As the show broke for a commercial, Juanita and her daughters entered the room.

> **Clinical Sidebar 8.5**
> For patients with significantly delayed word-finding behavior, rapid naming exercises may be helpful. The procedure is to provide pictures of familiar objects in rapid succession and encourage the patient to name them more rapidly. What other types of exercises might you use for rapid naming?

Juanita was dressed casually for the car trip and gave her ex-husband a parting kiss. But it was Johnny's daughters, ages 3, 5, and 7, who brought tears to the eyes of the rehabilitation nurse who was adjusting the bed sheets. They hugged and kissed him and promised never to forget him, but Johnny showed no emotion and said nothing. He continued to stare at the television set, apparently oblivious. Finally, the farewells were complete and the visitors left. During the entire emotional farewell, Johnny barely acknowledged their existence, and seemed to be more interested in the muted television talk show. As they entered the elevator, the quiet in Johnny's room was broken by the barely intelligible words, "Don't go."

Case Study 8.6 Pediatric Traumatic Brain Injury After a Hit-and-Run Motor Vehicle Accident

COLLIN

On a beautiful Saturday morning, 6-year-old Collin and his older brother, Travis, hurriedly finished their breakfast and ran out the door. Collin had wrapped his new baseball glove around a softball, and overnight, a perfect pocket had been created in the mitt. Travis, a fifth grader, was going to hit a few ground balls to Collin and show him the finer points of baseball.

For Lindsay and her friends, it had been one of the best sleepovers ever. They had spent the whole night sharing secrets and giggling about clumsy, awkward boys. The girls knew they were far more mature than their male peers, and a driver's license was soon to be the ultimate symbol of maturity. Fifteen-year-old Lindsay had just received her driver's permit, allowing her to drive as long as a licensed driver was present.

She hoped her parents would return from the restaurant they owned in time for her to drive her best friend home. Although the restaurant didn't open until 4:00 p.m., there were morning bread and produce deliveries to be inventoried. Lindsay's friend offered to call her parents for the ride home, but on this Saturday morning, the two girls made a bad decision. They thought that just this once, Lindsay would drive her friend home without a licensed adult in the car. It was a short drive. No one would be the wiser; besides, she was nearly a legal driver.

Collin was already showing promise as a shortstop; he had the necessary instinct and moves. Travis threw a ground ball, and Collin scrambled to capture it. After about an hour, Travis thought it time to hit a few grounders. He tossed the ball above his head, and as it fell he slammed the bat into it, sending it bouncing to Collin. So far, Collin had caught or stopped each ball. Then Travis hit a "zinger"; it bounced twice and shot over Collin's head, between the parked cars, and into the quiet street. Collin ran after it.

Lindsay carefully backed the family's second car out of the garage, down the driveway, and into the street. Just as the driving instructor had taught, she had her hands at 10 and 2 o'clock on the steering wheel. The two girls talked and laughed as the car came to a complete stop at the first stop sign. Looking both ways, Lindsay turned right and continued the short journey to her friend's house. The car accelerated to the speed limit, and then Lindsay briefly looked down to change the radio station. The police report listed the accident as a hit-and-run because the panicked and distraught girls, screaming and sobbing, had returned home.

Clinical Sidebar 8.6
A young child with traumatic brain injury is believed to have a better prognosis than an adult. Because of limited learning and experience, the youngster has a more "uncommitted cortex" than an adult, and it is more likely that other areas of the brain will take over for the damaged ones. Do you believe that the types of injuries suffered by children also affect their progress? What other factors might account for children having a better prognosis than adults?

Collin lay in the pediatric head trauma unit, with bandages around his head and tubes coming from his nose, wrist, and head. The room was dimly lighted, with several instruments humming and beeping. One instrument attached to Collin's arm monitored his blood pressure, and the frequency and strength of each heartbeat were displayed above the pressure reading. A pulse oximeter attached to his index finger provided valuable information about respiration and blood oxygen. The drainage tube attached to his head allowed a red-yellow fluid to fill a small bulb, reducing the pressure in his brain.

Several days later, Collin's parents accompanied him to the hospital's radiology unit for several diagnostic tests. The magnetic resonance imaging brain scans had helped to identify the site of Collin's brain injury. The front bumper of Lindsay's car had damaged primarily the frontal-temporal-parietal lobes of the left hemisphere. The pediatric neurologist told Collin's parents that those areas are all-important for speech and language. She was extremely pessimistic about his future ability to talk, walk, and take care of himself.

Five years have passed since Collin ran into the street chasing the errant baseball. The passage of time has been good for Travis and Lindsay. Travis no longer feels guilty about hitting the baseball too hard for a 6-year-old, and Lindsay, with the help of counseling and the kindness of Collin's parents, forgave herself for making bad decisions that Saturday morning. Finally, the brain's remarkable compensation abilities have been very good to Collin.

Collin is now in sixth grade, and with the help of resource teachers and speech, physical, and occupational therapists, he is learning, walking, and performing other activities of daily living very well. He goes to the resource room for special teaching and help with course assignments. The physical therapist works on improving the range of motion in his right leg, arm, and hand, and the occupational therapist has discovered clever new ways for Collin to button shirts, secure belts, and tie shoes. The latest neuropsychological and communication tests show the power of a young brain to compensate for bad baseball and driving judgments. Most of Collin's communication abilities are at age level, and on the tests of receptive vocabulary, that is, understanding words and their meanings, he scored higher than his peers. On Saturdays, Collin is the neighborhood team's shortstop. Now as a left hander, he can hit the baseball into the right field, where the opposing team puts its most awkward player. Collin is batting a thousand.

Case Study 8.7 Closed Head Injury Resulting from a Motorcycle Accident

PATIENT FOUR STAR

"He loves football," the young nurse says, "and we leave the sports channel on all the time." A man in his early 20s lies on the hospital bed staring at the television screen. He is tanned, muscular, clean-shaven, and looks as though he had stepped out of a surfboard advertisement. " **** " is listed for his name on the medical chart. It is hospital practice for four stars to be given when the patient is a public figure whose real name is to be kept confidential. It is also used when the patient is a suspect in a major crime or a witness to it and guards are stationed outside the room. But Patient Four Star, as he is called by the medical staff, is neither a public figure nor a crime boss; he is simply an unfortunate motorcycle accident victim with no identification. According to the records, he has been in the hospital for more than 2 months, and all attempts to identify him have been unsuccessful.

Early one morning, Patient Four Star and his crumpled motorcycle were discovered in a ravine. No one knows how long he had been unconscious or what caused the accident. Apparently, the high-powered motorcycle had been stolen, and the rider, helmetless and wearing only jeans, a sweatshirt, and expensive running shoes, was found 90 feet away and nearly out of sight of the police. He had no identification, or perhaps a thief had seen the accident and stolen it. Patient Four Star's fingerprints were run through every data bank in the state, his picture was shown on television newscasts, and a local private detective was hired to identify him. But it was to no avail; the true identity of Patient Four Star remained unknown. As a last-ditch effort, the hospital administrators and the county authorities, who are now

Clinical Sidebar 8.7
Hospital staff commonly leave the television on in the patient's room in the belief that it will provide the comatose or stuporous patient with needed stimulation. However, television programs consist of laugh tracks and artificial conversations that can further confuse the patient. They also can desensitize the patient to the speech of visitors and medical staff and compete for the patient's attention. Can you study better with the television on and with other distractions? Why can some students study with many distractions, whereas others are hindered by them?

responsible for him, have asked you to help. You are authorized to see Patient Four Star and try to get him to volunteer his name or other vital information. The neurologists and neuropsychologists think it a long shot but one worth pursuing. After all, the nurses report that he is becoming more aware and that he particularly likes watching the sports channel.

The chart shows that Patient Four Star has suffered a massive closed head injury. He is listed as being in an "eye-open vegetative state" and "decerebrate." An eye-open vegetative state is a condition of complete absence of awareness of the self; the patient is oblivious to the environment but has wake-sleep cycles. According to the medical reports, Patient Four Star awakens in the morning and opens his eyes; at night, he goes through the usual stages of sleep seen in normal persons. If you watch him sleep, you can see the rapid eye movements under his eyelids and the deep breathing as he apparently dreams. A decerebrate patient lacks higher level brain functions due to widespread cortical brain damage. Patient Four Star, like many decerebrate patients, occasionally has rigid extension of his limbs and lies in bed in this forced posture. On this rainy day in October, he is apparently captivated by the college football game.

"Where to begin?" you wonder as you pull up a chair and sit by Patient Four Star's bed. He is still focused on the football game halted by a timeout. You review the neurological report that was done several weeks ago. Perhaps some spontaneous recovery has occurred and the patient has improved. Just as the nurse observed, he seems to be an enthusiastic sports fan. Patient Four Star just might have a normal mind trapped in a spastic body. You have heard stories of such persons. You have seen movies of patients snapping out of comas after years of existing in an unconscious netherworld.

The neurological report shows that the patient does not startle to loud sounds or visually track. He does not anticipate a needle prick. According to the medical reports, Patient Four Star does not respond to any visual or verbal commands or internal needs. The coma scale places him almost at the lowest level compatible with survival. But he watches the televised football game with the same concentration as millions of sports fans. You wonder if he is irritated by your presence. When you shuffle the chart's paper, you expect him to turn up the sound and "shush" you. You suspect that the nurse was right; Patient Four Star is ready to tell his story.

The storm intensifies, and icy raindrops sound like sand hitting the window. The game has resumed. Then suddenly, the hospital lights flicker and the television's cable connection is broken. The picture dissolves, the announcer's voice becomes static noise, and the television screen turns to snow. You look at Patient Four Star and see that he is watching the snowy screen and listening to the noise with the same interest as he did the football game, and realize the futility of your assignment.

Case Study **8.8**   Closed Head Injury Resulting from an Airplane Accident

MARY LYNN PRITCHER

After graduating from an Ivy League university with a degree in recreational management, Mary Lynn Pritcher landed a job with the Department of the Interior. There she approved and monitored concession contracts for the Grand Canyon and Yellowstone National Parks. Selling hot dogs, bread, ice cream, and trinkets of wolves and geysers are big businesses in national parks, and she was responsible for tracking them. These restaurants and general stores turn big profits during the 3 or 4 months of the busy tourist season, and Mary Lynn's job was to make spot checks to ensure that tourists were treated fairly. This included unannounced site visits, and it was during one of them that her airplane crashed.

The Grand Canyon Airport is sizable enough for large passenger jets, but most of the aircraft taking off and landing are small single-engine planes. Much of the traffic at this tower-controlled airport involves six-passenger tour airplanes that fly scenic routes over the canyon. First, the airplanes fly west to majestic waterfalls. At the bottom of the canyon is a quaint village that is accessible only by foot, mule, or helicopter. Then the tour airplanes bank sharply and turn east, giving the passengers a clear view of the mile-deep canyon. They crisscross the 12-mile-wide expanse of the high desert canyon until they reach Glen Canyon Dam, Lake Powell, and its 100-mile shoreline. Then they again turn west, fly over the northern section of the largest stand of Ponderosa pine trees in the world, and return to the airport.

Several times in the past, Mary Lynn had taken rushed trips to the Grand Canyon National Park to spot check the concessionaires' compliance. Today she had some extra time and decided to take a scenic tour. The young pilot greeted them and announced that they would be having a great adventure, seeing one of the natural wonders of the world. He then notified the tower of his intent to depart, taxied to the end of the runway, again contacted the tower, and received permission to take off. The airplane began moving down the runway. It gradually accelerated, and soon its three wheels lifted off the pavement. When it was about 50 feet above the trees, an intense warning siren and a computer-generated voice from the instrument panel saying "Stall, stall, stall" were heard by the pilot and passengers. Then came a terrifying loud crash and a dense billow of black smoke rising above the tress.

Mary Lynn was treated first at the Grand Canyon Hospital and then flown by helicopter to a regional trauma center in Las Vegas, Nevada. Surgeons stopped the bleeding inside her brain and evacuated a large hematoma. During the crash, Mary Lynn had also suffered a broken neck, requiring a tracheotomy and a respirator for breathing. After surgery, she was transferred to the intensive care unit. Two weeks

Clinical Sidebar 8.8
A tracheotomy tube is placed in a patient's neck below the vocal cords, usually between the third and fourth tracheal rings. It allows air to enter the lungs and bypasses the larynx and upper air passageways. A *cuff* is a balloon-like structure surrounding the lower part of the tube; when inflated, it helps prevent food and liquid from entering the respiratory passageways. A fenestrated tracheotomy tube has a window cut into it to allow airflow for speech. What is the difference between a tracheotomy and a laryngectomy?

later, she was moved to the intermediate intensive care unit and later to a regular hospital room. About 3 weeks after the crash, Mary Lynn began to regain consciousness. She was then transferred to a rehabilitation hospital in Colorado specializing in traumatic head and neck injuries.

Mary Lynn spent nearly 1 year in the hospital. Her broken neck healed, and she was gradually weaned from the respirator. Fortunately, her spinal cord had not been completely severed during the accident, and she gradually regained partial sensation and motor function. Upon discharge from the hospital, she could walk with assistance for a short distance. With her left hand, she could control her motorized wheelchair and feed herself using specially designed utensils, plates, and cups. After many months of therapy, Mary Lynn could produce intelligible speech, although certain sounds were distorted, particularly those requiring elevation of the tongue. Tube feeding was discontinued, and eventually she was able to suck, chew, and swallow safely as long as meals were chopped and blended and liquids were thickened.

The right hemisphere and other parts of Mary Lynn's brain had been damaged, causing blindness on the left side of both eyes. The blindness, homonymous hemianopsia, was in the same visual half-field of both eyes. In Mary Lynn's case, it was left-homonymous hemianopsia, affecting the left side of her visual world. She also suffered from visual neglect, and initially did not cross the visual midline and attend to persons or things on the left side. When eating, Mary Lynn consumed only the foods on the right side of the plate, and when she applied makeup, it was only to the right side of her face. The visual field cut also affected her ability to read and name objects. Due to the right hemisphere brain damage, she also had problems appreciating facial expressions and interpreting verbal intent and emotion. Therapy was very helpful, and ultimately, when Mary Lynn was discharged to the specially designed apartment complex associated with the rehabilitation hospital, her communication abilities were functional and nearly normal.

SUMMARY

When an object impacts or penetrates a human brain, the results can be devastating to the patient and his or her family. Some patients are permanently comatose and spend the remainder of their lives oblivious to family and friends. Others gradually emerge from the coma and resume their lives, although with memory, learning, behavioral, and communication disorders. Some patients make a complete recovery, and go on to lead normal lives. Health care professionals come into these patients' lives at a very important time. Their knowledge, skill, and concern are powerful determinants of the patient's ultimate recovery.

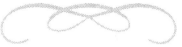

Study and Discussion Questions

1. What is the difference between closed and open head injury?

2. What is a coma? What are some diagnostic terms for and definitions of reduced awareness?

3. What is the difference between anterograde and retrograde amnesia?

4. Describe the types of neurogenic communication disorders resulting from traumatic brain injury.

5. How are memory and orientation related?

6. What is response delay?

7. Describe the lingering psychological and communication problems that may result from traumatic brain injury.

8. How might aphasic paraphasias cause the misdiagnosis of posttraumatic psychosis?

9. Compare and contrast the behavioral, emotional, cognitive, and communication impairments in pediatric and adult traumatic brain injury. What role does the patient's age play in determining the prognosis? Why is age a factor?

10. What types of tracheostomies exist, and how might they affect speech production?

Recommended Reading

Curran, C. A., Ponsford, J. L., & Crowe, S. (2000). Coping strategies and emotional outcomes following traumatic brain injury: A comparison with orthopedic patients. *Journal of Head Trauma Rehabilitation, 15*(6), 1256–1274.

   This article examines coping strategies and emotional outcomes in traumatic brain-injured patients.

Gillis, R., & Pierce, J. (1996). Mechanism of traumatic brain injury and the pathophysiologic consequences. In R. Gillis (Ed.), *Traumatic brain injury rehabilitation for speech-language pathologists* (pp. 38–54). Boston: Butterworth-Heinemann.

   This chapter provides a comprehensive review of traumatic brain injuries, communication disorders, and their treatment.

Tanner, D. (2003). *The psychology of neurogenic communication disorders: A primer for health care professionals.* Boston: Allyn & Bacon.

   This book examines neurogenic communication disorders, including those caused by traumatic brain injuries, and discusses coping styles and defense mechanisms.

Yeates, K. (2000). Closed-head injury. In K. Yeates, M. Ris, & H. Taylor (Eds.), *Pediatric neuropsychology* (pp. 92–116). New York: Guilford.

   This chapter discusses pediatric closed head injury.

CHAPTER NINE

Hearing Loss and Deafness

Silence is as full of potential wisdom and wit as the unhewn marble of great sculpture.

Aldous Huxley

Chapter Preview: This chapter examines the effects of hearing loss and deafness on the ability to communicate. There is an overview of the hearing mechanism and the associated energy transformations. Etiologies of hearing loss and deafness are reviewed, as are screening and site of lesion testing. Technological advances in amplification and cochlear implants, as well as their social implications, are critiqued. Some case studies address industrial hearing testing, deafness and meningitis, and presbycusis. Others focus on a cochlear implant, the social aspects of deafness, and hearing loss associated with traumatic brain injury.

OVERVIEW OF AUDIOLOGY, HEARING LOSS, AND DEAFNESS

Audiology, the science of hearing and the diagnosis and non-medical treatment of hearing loss, is a rapidly evolving profession. It developed after World War II as an independent clinical discipline because of the large number of soldiers with noise-induced hearing loss (Martin, 1997). The American Speech-Language-Hearing Association and the American Academy of Audiology, two professional organizations for audiologists, have established the academic requirements and scope of practice for their members.

Audiologists are distinct from hearing aid dispensers. Hearing aid dispensers, formerly called *hearing aid audiologists,* have limited education and training in the diagnosis and management of hearing loss and deafness. The term currently preferred by the International Hearing Society, and by many state licensure boards, is *hearing instrument specialist.* However, most audiologists can also dispense hearing aids. Currently, the terminal degree for audiologists is the master's degree, but soon it will be the clinical doctorate (AuD). Audiologists are becoming increasingly involved in **aural rehabilitation**, the development and integration of residual hearing to maximize auditory perception. Aural rehabilitation also includes educational techniques to improve expression. Speech-language pathologists and audiologists overlap in the clinical management of persons with

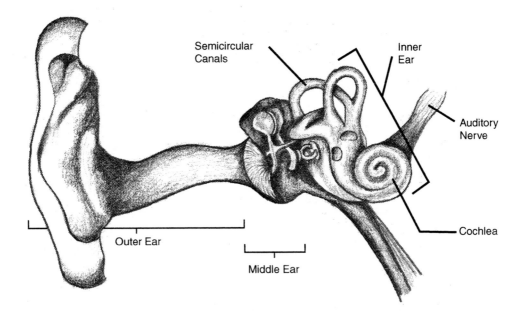

Semicircular
Canals

Inner
Ear

Auditory
Nerve

Cochlea

Outer Ear

Middle Ear

Figure 9.1 Major landmarks of the outer, middle, and inner ears.

hearing loss and **deafness.** Hearing loss is the reduced ability to sense sound, and deafness denotes the inability to perceive sound with or without amplification. Sometimes, the term **hard-of-hearing** is used to refer to hearing loss and deafness.

Hearing is sometimes called the *second sense,* after vision, in transmitting knowledge of the world. However, when it comes to the acquisition of speech, hearing is primary and vital. For example, a child born deaf will not naturally acquire the ability to speak, and a child born with a hearing loss will have speech that reflects the frequency and severity of the loss. Besides its importance for speech communication, hearing conveys the sounds of the environment. It brings persons in constant contact with reality, alerting them to enjoyment and danger.

Anatomy and Physiology of the Hearing Mechanism

As Figure 9.1 demonstrates, the human ear can be separated into **outer, middle,** and **inner** sections. The external ear directs the acoustic energy generated by the sound source into the **ear canal,** which is covered by a waxy secretion, **cerumen,** that protects it. The ear canal is a self-cleaning structure; it is not necessary to remove cerumen in most persons. In the middle ear, acoustic energy is transformed into mechanical energy. The **tympanic membrane,** or eardrum, vibrates in response to the vibrations of the air particles in the ear canal. The smallest bones in the human body, the **ossicles,** which are connected to the tympanic membrane, amplify the energy and direct it to the **cochlea.** The ossicles are the

malleus, incus, and **stapes,** also known as the *hammer, anvil,* and *stirrup,* respectively. The middle ear is a small chamber ventilated by the **eustachian tube,** which acts to equalize middle ear and atmospheric pressure. Mechanical energy from the middle ear is transformed into hydraulic energy in the inner ear, consisting of the **semicircular canals** and the cochlea. The semicircular canals are part of the vestibular mechanism and are important for balance. The hydraulic vibrations in the cochlea are transformed into electrochemical or nerve energy at the **vestibulo-cochlear cranial nerve** (VIII), or auditory nerve, and sent to higher brain centers, where auditory perception and association occur.

Categories of Hearing Loss

There are three general categories of hearing loss: **conductive, sensorineural,** and **mixed.** Conductive hearing loss results from impaired functioning of the external or middle ear. Sensorineural hearing loss is due to impaired functioning of the cochlea or cranial nerve VIII. Mixed hearing loss involves both conductive and sensorineural components. In addition, **auditory processing disorders** concern perception and association of auditory stimuli due to neurological damage or abnormalities in the brainstem or higher cortical levels. Each is discussed in detail below.

Typical Causes of Hearing Loss and Deafness

Otitis media is the most common cause of conductive hearing loss in children. *Otitis* refers to inflammation, and *media* indicates its location at the level of the middle ear. (**Otitis externa,** also known as *swimmer's ear,* is inflammation of the external ear.) Often in otitis media, the eustachian tube does not equalize pressure between the middle ear and the external atmosphere. In middle ear infections, the tympanic membrane does not function properly and may rupture. A **myringotomy tube** can be placed in the tympanic membrane to equalize pressure.

Recently, there has been controversy about the placement of myringotomy tubes; some pediatricians believe they are unnecessary, easily dislodged, and have little medical benefit. By contrast, some otologists believe they reduce symptoms and prevent hearing loss. Otitis media also occurs in adults, but **otosclerosis,** calcification and fixation of the ossicles, is another frequent cause of conductive hearing loss. Other causes of conductive hearing loss include prolonged impacted cerumen, narrowing (stenosis) of the external ear canal, and trauma.

Sensorineural hearing loss is frequently caused by excessive and prolonged exposure to noise. Noise-induced hearing loss may also occur as a result of sudden loud noises such as gunshots, bombs, and industrial explosions. The terms **barotrauma** and **acoustic trauma** are sometimes used to refer to hearing loss due to sudden explosive noise. "As a rule, the amounts of hearing loss are similar in both ears when individuals acquire noise-induced hearing losses in the workplace. Rifle shooters generally show more hearing loss in the ear opposite the shoulder to which the rifle stock is held, that is, right-handed shooters will have more hearing loss in the left ear" (Martin & Clark, 2003, p. 298). Other causes of sensorineural hearing loss include **toxins, meningitis, presbycusis,** a progressive hearing loss in both ears occurring with aging, and **Meniere's disease**, a sudden disorder of the inner ear characterized by tinnitus and progressive low-frequency hearing loss. Meniere's disease is also associated with dizziness and nausea and can be considered a syndrome.

Mixed hearing loss can result from combinations of the above conductive and sensorineural etiological factors. Traditionally, the hallmark of mixed hearing loss is **depressed air and bone conduction thresholds** and the **air-bone gap** discussed in the section Audiograms and Types of Hearing Loss.

Tumors, trauma, strokes, aging, and disease processes can cause auditory processing disorders, and because definitions of the nature and symptoms of different disorders vary, the etiology of many cases is idiopathic. The term *auditory processing disorders,* formerly referred to as *central auditory processing disorders,* is a vague diagnostic label and can include auditory and acoustic agnosia. When addressed by an audiologist, auditory processing disorders are part of aural habilitation or rehabilitation; when considered by a speech-language pathologist, they are a component of agnosia or aphasia therapy.

Tinnitus

Tinnitus is usually described as the sensation of ringing in the ear. A more precise definition is the sensation of noise in the head without external stimulation through the ear. The noise can also be described as buzzing, whistling, roaring, and so forth. The condition is associated with damage to the hearing mechanism as a result of noise exposure, toxins, disease, hypertension, and several other factors. For some persons, tinnitus is a minor nuisance; for others, it can be a major disability significantly affecting the quality of life. Unfortunately, although there are several medical and behavioral treatments for tinnitus, little can be done to eliminate it.

Audiograms and Types of Hearing Loss

Audiograms are graphic representations of hearing test results. They provide a visual depiction of the person's hearing **thresholds** and serve as a basis for interpreting audiometric results. The test frequencies are listed in **hertz** (Hz) along the top and the patient's hearing level in **decibels** (dB) down the left side. Air conduction test results are plotted at the intersection of the frequency and decibel lines using 0 markings for the right ear and X markings for the left ear. In **bone conduction** test results, "<" represents the right ear and ">" the left one. Bone conduction bypasses the external and middle ears and transmits sound through the bones of the head. Because of cross-hearing, sometimes it is necessary to perform **masking**, that is, to introduce a competing sound during the test. Masked symbols are "[" and "]" for the right and left ears, respectively.

Figure 9.2 presents an audiogram of a binaural conductive hearing loss. It shows similar depressed pure tone air conduction thresholds in the 30- to 40-dB range with no discernible slope. Bone conduction testing reveals normal thresholds. Together, air and bone conduction results depict a typical air-bone gap. This audiogram shows the patient's ability to hear better through bone conduction than air conduction, indicating that the lesion is located in the external or middle ear.

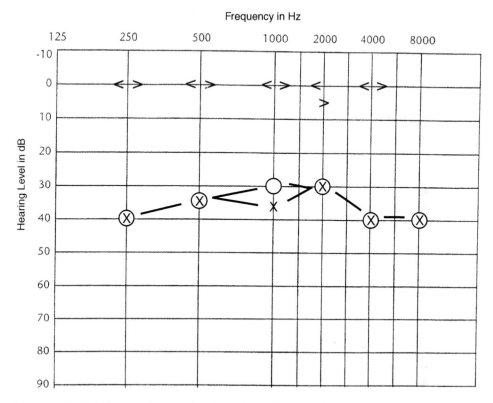

Figure 9.2 Binaural conductive hearing loss.

Figure 9.3 shows a binaural sensorineural hearing loss. In this audiogram, bone and air conduction thresholds are depressed in both ears, with gradually decreasing hearing sensitivity in the 2000-, 4000-, and 8000-Hz ranges. In mixed hearing loss, bone conduction thresholds are also depressed.

Acoustic Impedance Audiometry and Middle-Ear Testing

According to Martin and Clark (2003, p. 144), the common use of the term **impedance audiometry** is technically incorrect: "Because audiometry per se is involved only with respect to the acoustic reflex, this term is not strictly accurate." They also note that referencing this type of testing to the middle ear is misleading because it primarily involves the tympanic membrane, not direct testing of the entire middle ear. However, because of their widespread acceptance by clinicians from a variety of disciplines, the terms *acoustic impedance audiometry* and *middle-ear testing* are used rather than more technically accurate terms such as *acoustic immittance metering*. Typically, acoustic impedance audiometry provides three measurements of middle-ear functioning: **compliance**, **stapedial reflex**, and **tympanometry**.

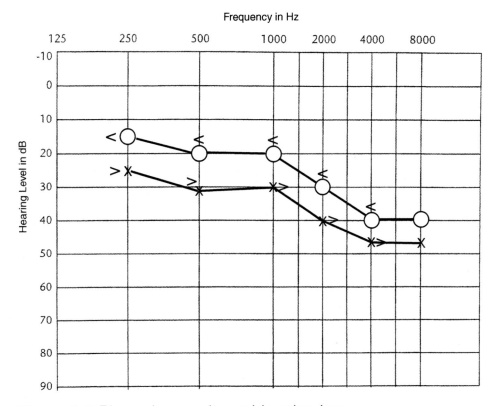

Figure 9.3 Binaural sensorineural hearing loss.

In audiometry, compliance is the ease with which the middle ear structures function. Technically, static acoustic compliance indicates the flexibility and mobility of the middle ear structures, particularly the tympanic membrane. Stapedial reflex refers to the protective action of the stapedius muscle (and tensor tympani) in response to loud sounds. The stapes, the smallest bone of the ossicular chain, is in contact with the **oval window** of the cochlea. The contraction of this muscle protects the ear by increasing the impedance of the middle ear and thus reducing the potential damage caused by loud sounds. Tympanometry measures the middle ear pressure changes and the compliance of the tympanic membrane in response to pressure changes due to the testing device. The presence or absence of the stapedial reflex, positive and negative pressures, and increased or reduced compliance provides diagnostic information about the functioning of the tympanic membrane, eustachian tubes, and ossicular chain.

Speech Audiometry

According to Martin and Clark (2003), the terminology for **speech audiometry** has been inconsistent. In general, speech audiometry consists of measuring a patient's ability to hear and understand syllables and words. The stimuli control for stress and use **phonetically balanced words**, monosyllables with the same distribution of phonemes occurring in connected speech. Specific **speech recognition** and **discrimination testing** is done to determine the patient's minimum intensity levels required to detect speech and discriminate words. Speech audiometry also addresses the patient's loudness comfort level.

Newborns, Infants, and Hard-to-Test Populations

It is vitally important to detect hearing loss and deafness in children as early as possible. A child with unidentified significant hearing loss or deafness suffers psychologically, educationally, and socially. One way of testing newborns, infants, and hard-to-test populations (e.g., mentally retarded, with reduced consciousness, or demented) is behavioral: examining actions such as the head turning, startle reflex, or sucking behavior of the infant or child in response to auditory stimuli. Technological advances have dramatically improved newborn and infant hearing screening procedures. "The conventional methods for audiological evaluations of infants and young children are **otoacoustic emissions** (OAE), **behavioral testing** and **tympanometry**. These procedures also can be used for pediatric populations with special needs, but modifications may be required" (Klimas, 2003, p. 23). Klimas notes that **auditory brainstem responses** (ABRs) may be measured while the patient is sedated and can be useful for difficult populations who cannot be tested behaviorally.

OAEs are sounds emanating from the external ear as a result of cochlear vibration. According to Martin and Clark (2003), there are two classes of OAE: **spontaneous** and **transient-evoked** (TEOAE). Spontaneous OAEs occur in over one half of persons with normal hearing and thus have little diagnostic significance. TEOAEs are produced by brief stimuli such as clicks. "When a TEOAE is not seen, the suggestion is that a hearing loss is present, but does not reveal whether the problem is in the conductive pathway or the cochlea" (Martin & Clark, 2003, p. 159). Yellin, Culbertson, Tanner, and Adams (2000a, 2000b) report the use of TEOAEs for early hearing screening in a well-baby nursery and note that gender differences exist among newborns.

ABR testing, sometimes called **brainstem evoked response audiometry** (BSER), is a test of the auditory system in which repetitive sounds such as clicks are used as stimuli. ABR is one of several objective electrophysiological auditory tests that measure the neural activity of the auditory system. During ABR testing, the brief repetitive sounds produce electrical activity along the auditory system, providing information about the site of a lesion.

Hearing Aids

Digital hearing aids have dramatically improved the quality of amplification for hearing-impaired individuals. The increased quality of digital technology compared to earlier analog hearing aids can be likened to the improved musical quality of compact disks over vinyl records. However, in spite of this new technology, no hearing aid provides the clarity, distinctness, naturalness, and clearness of speech and environmental sounds of the normal ear. Consequently, many people with hearing loss are disappointed when their hearing is not returned to normal.

In general, three types of hearing aids exist: **body**, **eyeglasses**, and **ear**. In the body hearing aid, the battery power and associated equipment are carried in a specially constructed body pack or in a pocket of the person's clothing. This hearing aid reduces the high-pitched feedback that is troublesome to many hearing aid wearers. Because there is less miniaturization, the controls are more easily adjusted to different sound environments, and large headphones can be used. An added advantage of body hearing aids is that a teacher can use a microphone and talk to several children wearing these devices.

Eyeglass hearing aids are more comfortable for some wearers than those positioned behind or in the ear. However, they have several disadvantages. First, because the electronics are built into the eyeglass temple positioning arm, when the person requires new eyeglasses, the hearing aid or aids must also be replaced. Second, hearing aids are usually worn most of the time, whereas many persons wear glasses only for reading or driving. Third, many eyeglass hearing aids have large temple positioning arms and tend to be unfashionable.

There are two general varieties of ear hearing aids: **behind-the-ear** and **in-the-ear** (Other descriptive terms are *full shell, half shell, canal, mini-canal,* and *completely-in-the-canal,* the name indicating the location of the electronic equipment.) Behind-the-ear hearing aids were once the type most often used. These aids are obtrusive, and many hard-of-hearing persons refuse to wear devices that draw attention to their disorder. Because of improved miniaturization and digital technology, in-the-ear (partial or complete) hearing aids now provide almost invisible aided hearing. An added advantage of in-the-ear and completely-in-the-ear hearing aids is that there is less wind noise since the microphone is seated within the ear canal (Mueller & Carter, 2002).

Cochlear Implants

The first human **cochlear implant** occurred in 1972; initially, it was available only to adults with profound acquired hearing loss (Nelson, 2000). Now it is provided to children and adults meeting the guidelines of the Food and Drug Administration (FDA). According to Nelson (2000), candidates must have bilateral profound sensorineural hearing loss (adults may have bilateral severe to profound hearing loss if acquired after the development of speech and language), limited or no useful benefit from hearing aids, and no medical contraindications. Children and their caregivers must have high motivation, realistic expectations, and educational placement that emphasizes auditory skills development. Children must be at least 18 months of age and adults at least 17 years old.

The cochlear implant allows direct stimulation of the auditory nerve. The internal receiver, consisting of wire electrodes placed in the **scala tympani** within the cochlea, is implanted under the skin (Martin & Clark, 2003). Holmes (2002) describes the surgery:

> The cochlear implant surgery is completed under general anesthesia. Typically, the surgeon makes an incision behind the ear and drills a small area in the mastoid bone for the placement of the receiver simulator and the insertion of the electrode array. The electrode array is then threaded through the mastoid and the middle ear cavity and then inserted in the scala tympani of the cochlea through the round window. Insertion depths can range up to 30 mm depending on the implant system being used. The operation normally ranges from 1 to 3 hours and often is done on an outpatient basis. (p. 82)

After surgery, the patient receives aural habilitation or rehabilitation to maximize the implant's benefits. The costs of cochlear implants and related services are usually covered by major insurance carriers and Medicare. In some states, Medicaid and Vocational Rehabilitation Services also cover these costs (Holmes, 2002).

Aural Habilitation and Rehabilitation

The concepts of **habilitation** and **rehabilitation**, although related, differ technically. Habilitation is the development of a person's function or the ability to perform normally or near-normally. Rehabilitation is the restoration of function, after a disorder or disease, to normal or near-normal status. For the deaf neonate, aural habilitation involves the development of optimal existing communication abilities. For the youngster or adult who becomes deaf or hard-of-hearing after having functional hearing, aural rehabilitation consists of the effective use of **residual** hearing, including the memory of audition, as a catalyst for optimal communication. Although the objectives are similar, relearning a function after having lost it is different from learning a new one for the first time. Because of the technical differences between aural habilitation and rehabilitation, the following discussion is separated into services for children and adults.

Approaches for Children

Three variables directly affect aural habilitation and rehabilitation in children. First, some hearing losses and deafness are **congenital**, that is, apparent at birth. "Youngsters with congenital deafness should generally be served through early-intervention programs, which include parent-infant and preschool programs" (Moellar, Schow, & Johnson, 2002, p. 279). Second, some hearing loss and deafness may occur after birth, but before or during the major speech and language acquisition period. In these cases, the age at which the disorder takes place and the child's level of speech and language acquisition dictate the nature and type of aural rehabilitation services provided. The child can be seen in early-intervention programs, in the school, and in other clinical settings. Third, some hearing loss and deafness may occur after speech and language development, roughly after the age of 8 years. According to the IDEA, children with hearing loss must receive free, appropriate educational services in the least restrictive environment. Although vocabulary and pragmatics are learned throughout life, most children have learned language and phonemes by age 7 or 8 (Tanner, Culbertson, & Secord, 1997; Tanner, Lamb & Secord, 1997).

According to Nicolosi, Harryman, and Kresheck (2004), all aural habilitation and rehabilitation is based on two methodologies: **analytic** and **synthetic**. The analytic, or formal, method emphasizes learning the parts of speechreading (lipreading) before addressing them holistically. In this method, the clinician teaches the hard-of-hearing or deaf person to recognize the speech sounds in isolation, later progressing to words, phrases, sentences, and longer units. In this approach to speechreading, the prosodic aspects are emphasized (Jena method), including rapid and rhythmic drills (Mueller-Walle method) and close observation of the movement of the lips from one sound position to another (Bruhn method). The synthetic, or informal, method addresses the meaning of whole paragraphs before breaking them into smaller units. This approach to speechreading emphasizes the intuition, quickness, concentration, and alertness of the speechreader in dealing with larger units prior to addressing words and sentences (Nitchie method).

Moellar et al. (2002) describe auditory skills for children. **Attending and detection** involve focusing on environmental sounds, voices, and distinct speech sounds. **Recognizing and locating** entail recognizing objects and events from their sounds and locating them in space. **Distance and levels** require localizing sound sources at increasing distances and "above and below." **Environmental discrimination**, **identification**, and **comprehension** consist of repeated stimulation with meaningful sounds to improve comprehension. **Vocal discrimination**, **identification**, and **comprehension** involve giving the child natural opportunities to distinguish onomatopoeic gross vocal sounds, words, and phrases. **Speech discrimination**, **identification**, and **comprehension** provide the child with opportunities to use these behaviors with meaningful fine speech sounds in words and in different situations. According to Moellar et al., these seven skills are not necessarily discrete stages; they form a general hierarchy with individual variations.

Articulation therapy for children with hearing loss requires special adaptations. The **sensorimotor method** is required rather than the phonological processes approach to articulation therapy for children with hearing loss (Waldowski & Wilkes, 2003). According to Waldowski and Wilkes, seven strategies can be used to improve articulation in children with hearing loss: working from the known to the unknown, using facilitating contexts, teaching by analogy, establishing a set, listening, analyzing errors, and providing specific feedback. After the child receives a hearing aid or cochlear implant, the feedback system provides a way of remembering sounds and connecting them to hearing.

School-age children who are deaf or hard-of-hearing require several adaptations in inclusive educational settings (Moellar et al., 2002). First, each child's communication strengths and weaknesses should be comprehensively evaluated. Second, intervention should address functioning in the classroom and those behaviors that lead to successful classroom listening. Third, new vocabulary words should be linked to existing knowledge. Fourth, narration focusing on organization and self-expression should be used to improve both oral and written communication. Fifth, verbal reasoning should be encouraged. Finally, according to Moellar et al., deaf and hard-of-hearing students benefit from the development of study skills and other classroom survival activities.

Approaches for Adults

Pichora-Fuller and Schow (2002) describe audiological rehabilitation management for hearing-impaired adults. These strategies follow a comprehensive assessment model that includes testing (see above) and self-reports. The primary audiological management strategies are summed up in the acronym CARE: **counseling**, **audibility** and instrumental interventions, **remediation** for communication activities, and **environmental** coordination and participation improvement.

Counseling addresses the factors that predispose, enable, and reinforce a hearing-impaired person's positive adjustment to the hearing loss. Audibility and instrumentation intervention applies to the fit and function of amplification devices including hearing aids, cochlear implants, and other assistive listening technologies. Remediation for communication activities involves the individual's behavioral changes in hearing-demanding activities to maximize the effects of amplification. Environmental coordination and participation improvement goals include ensuring that the person's social and physical environments support his or her participation in everyday life. According to Pichora-Fuller and Schow (2002), "In the management process, the rehabilitative audiologist works together with the individual with hearing loss and his or her communication partners to find a combination of solutions that will enable listening goals to be attained and maintained in a wide range of life circumstances" (p. 355).

Social Implications of Deafness

Controversy exists in the **deaf community** about whether deafness should be considered a disability and what types of habilitation and rehabilitation should be used by its members, particularly children. These issues often center on the **oralist, manualist**, and **total communication** philosophies. The oralists advocate developing speech and speechreading for communication purposes. Using residual hearing and undergoing extensive speech therapy and aural habilitation and rehabilitation, children learn to produce intelligible speech and to read the speech (lipread) of others. The speech of many individuals with little residual hearing often has a "hollow" and nasal characteristic. Although generally thought to be highly accurate, speechreading often provides far less than perfect understanding for the reader even when the speaker's lips and face are unobstructed. Comprehension is reduced because many speech sounds are produced in the back of the oral cavity and are not visible to the speech reader. Understanding sign language and using written communication can promote receptive communication. This approach also uses the person's residual hearing and amplification to produce the best speech possible. Advocates for the oralist approach note that being able to interact verbally increases the person's social and vocational opportunities.

Manualists believe that **American Sign Language** (ASL), is the natural and preferred language of the deaf community. ASL, a gestural form of communication, is a rich language unto itself. It meets the definition of language with its own unique grammar, syntax, and semantic representations. The role of language in developing and maintaining cultural and ethnic identity is critical, and ASL is an example of linguistic diversity. Manualists note the importance of adhering to the natural language of the community to give its members a sense of identity. The role of language in the human thought process also supports the manualists' advocacy of ASL for the deaf. Thinking in one language, using its arbitrary symbols and grammar, is different from thinking in another language, and the grammar and symbolic representations of ASL provide a unique cognitive perspective for the user.

The total communication approach integrates the oral and manual methods, maximizing the person's speechreading and residual hearing while teaching sign language. Proponents of this approach note that children taught by both the oral and manual methods can develop optimal abilities to interact with the hearing and verbal communities. Total communication also maximizes learning opportunities, and children can be mainstreamed.

Is deafness a disability or are persons who use manual communication a linguistic minority? Should profoundly hard-of-hearing and deaf children be taught only one method of aural habilitation or rehabilitation? Should these children be given cochlear implants and amplification? These are sensitive questions requiring respect for parents' and children's rights and the beliefs of some in the deaf community. However, technological, habilitative, and rehabilitative advances have dramatically changed those social and political issues. Cochlear implants, in particular, have created opportunities for persons to hear, although with individual variations in sound quality and speech discrimination abilities. The cochlear implant's ability to provide sound and speech sensation, perception, and discrimination has dramatically improved deaf and profoundly hard-of-hearing children's opportunities to communicate verbally. The cochlear implant is an evolving technology that will likely continue to improve the quantity and quality of hearing for these individuals. Hearing loss and deafness profoundly damage the person's present and future quality of life, especially reducing opportunities to learn. According to Northern and Downs (2002), a child with a severe hearing loss may incur a staggering economic cost over a lifetime: $2 million. Deafness is a disability, and to refuse to provide optimal habilitative and rehabilitative opportunities for deaf and profoundly hard-of-hearing persons is morally and ethically unacceptable. No one, including deaf and hard-of-hearing children, should be forced into a minority culture and deprived of the opportunity to interact freely with the larger verbal population. It should be noted that as children mature, they can choose to revert to manual communication alone and embrace the manualist deaf community (Tanner, 2003).

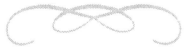

Case Studies in Hearing Loss and Deafness

Case Study 9.1 Industrial Hearing Testing and Noise-Induced Hearing Loss

INKOM NUCLEAR GENERATING PLANT

As someone who performs hearing testing in various industries, you have been taught about the role noise exposure plays in hearing loss and deafness, but nothing has prepared you for this practical lesson. You know about temporary threshold shifts and have even experienced them in loud bars and dance halls. You wear ear protection when shooting, riding motorcycles, and running the chainsaw to avoid permanent threshold shifts. You are aware of the havoc noise can wreak on hearing, but seeing worker after worker with the same type of audiogram drives home the noise–hearing loss lesson.

The Inkom Nuclear Generating Plant has more than 200 employees and many subcontractors. It is one of the largest generating plants in the nation, containing three large conical towers with steam billowing from the reactors. Hundreds of gallons of water are pumped into the facility each day to cool the nuclear reactor and to produce electricity with the large turbines. The turbines create a constant high-pitched scream as they convert nuclear energy into electricity. You drive your van and hearing testing trailer into the parking lot. Today you will test the hearing of the first shift of workers employed at various sites in the plant. The company nurse will assist you and has arranged the schedule. On this visit, each employee will receive a pure-tone evaluation.

The first group of employees to be tested is the security officers. Each employee enters the portable testing booth, and you place the earphones over his or her ears. First, you test 1000 Hz at 30 dB in the right ear. When the tone is heard, the employee raises a hand. Then you use the ascending-descending method, dropping the decibel level by 10 dB, doing this repeatedly until the employee no longer hears the tone. Next, you raise the level by 5 dB until the employee's hearing threshold at a particular frequency—the decibel level at which at least three out of the six presentations of the tone can be heard—is determined. After 1000 Hz is tested, you determine the hearing threshold for 2000, 4000, and 6000 Hz and then drop to the lowest frequencies: 125 and 250 Hz. After completing the test in the right ear, you use the same procedure in the left one. For every threshold obtained, you note the results on an audiogram: red circles for the right ear and blue Xs for the left one.

Clinical Sidebar 9.1

The *Lombard effect* is a speaker's natural tendency to increase the intensity of his or her voice when listening to a loud noise. The Lombard test is used to determine nonorganic hearing loss and malingering. Have you ever seen a person increase his or her voice level when talking while listening to music through headphones? Has this ever happened to you?

The next group of employees is from the turbine generating section—engineers, technicians, and mechanics who work behind a protective barrier, monitoring the turbine and cooling facilities. A constant high-pitched hum penetrates the protective walls of the section, requiring them to speak loudly or shout. When they enter the generating zone, they wear special ear protection. Many employees have worked in this noisy environment for several years.

Eventually, you test all three shifts of employees from the turbine generating section and, with few exceptions, find bilateral hearing loss in the higher frequencies. Some thresholds are more depressed than others, but a clear pattern of noise–induced hearing loss has emerged. Of course, there are many variables to consider before attributing the hearing loss to noise exposure in the workplace, including age, gender, and medical histories. You check each subject's employment file and find evidence that the longer an employee has worked in the generating section, the more depressed are his or her thresholds at 1000, 2000, 4000, and 8000 Hz. The hearing loss gradually increases in the higher frequencies.

Your audiological consulting company reviews the test results and investigates the sound levels and the length of time the employees of the turbine generating section are exposed to the noise. Sound level meters are used to measure the intensity of the noise emanating from the generators. The effectiveness of the employees' ear protection is investigated, as is the time each employee is exposed to extreme noise with and without ear protection. Several months later, the Inkom Nuclear Generating Plant enacts new regulations about noise and employees' duration of exposure, and purchases new, more effective, and more comfortable hearing protection. Supervisors also monitor employees' compliance with the new regulations.

Case Study 9.2   Meningitis and Deafness in a 5-Year-Old Girl

ILENE

Faculty and student eagerly anticipate the spring softball tournament. The faculty and their spouses proudly wear T-shirts labeled "Ossicles," and those of the students and their guests are marked "Speechies." The Audiology and Speech Sciences Department has sponsored this tournament and picnic for years. The events are held at the fairgrounds picnic area, usually in early May. This year it is unusually cold, with some rain, but the game and picnic proceed as scheduled. Of course children are welcome, but one them, 5-year-old Ilene, seems under the weather.

Clinical Sidebar 9.2
As a general rule, when talking to persons with a conductive hearing loss, speaking more loudly improves their understanding. When talking to persons with a sensorineural hearing loss, talking a little more loudly is often helpful and clearly articulating each speech sound is beneficial. What other things can speakers do to help a person with a hearing loss to understand their speech?

The softball game begins at 4:00. By 6:30, when it ends and the picnic begins, Ilene stands under a tree obviously cold, with watery eyes, sniffles, and complaining of an earache. Several persons offer her jackets and blankets. Her mother is concerned, and they leave early.

The next day, Ilene is admitted to the hospital's intensive care unit with the diagnosis of probable meningitis—inflammation of the membranes surrounding the brain and spinal cord. There are two types of this serious illness: bacterial and viral. The doctor believes that Ilene has the bacterial form, which is more common in young children. Ilene presented with acute onset of fever, headache, vomiting, earache, and a stiff neck. In the emergency room, she lost consciousness and suffered a seizure. Prompt, aggressive medical treatment probably saved Ilene's life but not her hearing. The doctor prepared Ilene's mother for the worst: about 20% of patients with bacterial meningitis can have partial or complete sensorineural hearing loss.

Several days later, an audiologist tests Ilene's hearing. The results confirm that she has suffered severe sensorineural damage to both ears. The audiologist's diagnosis is profound hearing loss because her pure tone hearing threshold averages are below 90 dB. And because Ilene is 5 years old, she is between two clinical definitions of deafness.

In the first definition, Ilene could be considered *adventitiously* or *prelingually deaf*. These individuals have not had functional hearing long enough to learn and use speech and language normally. However, because the acquisition of speech and language is a gradual process, the effects vary with the age at which the child becomes deaf. If deafness occurs after the acquisition of speech and language, the child has had functional hearing long enough to learn speech sounds and to develop the fabric of language. Sometimes the term *postlingual deafness* is used to refer to such persons. Because of Ilene's age, and because she learned speech and language early, she is placed in the postlingual deafness category. Sadly, the meningitis has damaged more than Ilene's hearing; her intelligence is also affected.

The audiologist gives Ilene a body-style hearing aid, which provides high levels of amplification and avoids the high-pitched feedback of many standard hearing aids producing maximum amplification. An added advantage is that the controls of the body hearing aid are large enough for her to adjust the volume easily in different learning environments. Ilene also learns to read lips and to express herself through a combination of speech and sign language.

Case Study **9.3**   **Hearing Loss in an 89-Year-Old Man**

IVAN

Ivan has lived through two world wars, the Korean and Vietnam conflicts, and the tragedy of September 11, 2001. He has seen the infancy of flight, witnessed landings on the moon, and viewed two space shuttle disasters. In his youth, he rode in horse-drawn buggies and black Model T and Model A jalopies. Now, in the sunset of his life, he rides in a car with satellite global positioning, an XM radio, a DVD screen, and On-Star telephone capabilities. In school, he learned to use the slide rule; now he occasionally surfs the Internet. During his working life as a farmer and rancher, he fed millions of Americans.

Noise has been a big part of Ivan's life. Farming and ranching have periods of quiet solitude, but too often they are noisy occupations. Tractors, a mainstay for the farmer and rancher, are loud machines. Early in Ivan's life, the tractor was a relatively quiet steel-wheeled three-wheeler coughing and choking through wheat, hay, and potato fields. Today it is a megamachine with huge wheels, an air-conditioned cab, power steering, and an engine capable of pulling a 10-point plow. Constant noise is a by-product of its power. Bailers, which turn rows of alfalfa into neat bales, are loud compressing and knot-tying contraptions. Hay choppers that pulverize the bales of hay into powder for cattle consumption nearly deafen anyone within earshot. Many factors may be responsible for Ivan's significant hearing loss, but decades of noise exposure are the prime culprit.

Like many persons suffering from gradual-onset hearing loss, Ivan denied it and engaged in projection. In his early 60s, he started having difficulty understanding the speech of family and

Clinical Sidebar 9.3
The loudness of environmental sounds varies dramatically. Normal breathing and a soft whisper are barely audible, at about 10–20 dB, while a jet airplane at takeoff can produce noise in excess of 150 dB. Bars and dance halls can produce extremely loud sounds and damage the hearing of musicians and patrons alike. Name the bars and dance halls where you live that produce the loudest sounds and possibly damage your hearing.

friends. Because the higher frequencies in the speech range were most impaired early on, he had particular difficulty understanding the speech of women and children, and often complained that they mumbled. As his hearing loss worsened progressively, he finally agreed to be tested for a hearing aid.

During the test, Ivan observed the examination of his external ear canal and eardrum on a video monitor. The audiologist performed a series of tests involving pure tones and pressure changes in his ear. A tape recording of *spondees,* words with two syllables produced with equal stress, was given to him, as were phonetically balanced words, to test his ability to receive and discriminate speech. The evaluation was conducted in a soundproof booth, and toward the end of testing, several aids were tried to determine which ones provided the best results.

The new digital hearing aids convert speech and environmental sounds into numbers and modify them. The amplified sound is then fed into the person's ears. Using them, Ivan was impressed by his improved ability to understand speech. It took several months before he became accustomed to them, and he was disappointed at their performance in environments with competing noise. However, they gradually became a part of his life and improved his ability to communicate with his loved ones.

Case Study **9.4** Idiopathic Progressive Hearing Loss and Cochlear Implant

TOAST

"Toast," as Ryan was nicknamed by his friends, started coming to the university speech and hearing clinic in his early teens. The audiologists could not determine the cause of his rapidly deteriorating hearing. Toast and his family took several trips to the Mayo Clinic in Rochester, Minnesota, to be evaluated and diagnosed, but the specialists all described the origin of his hearing loss the same way: idiopathic. There were many theories about why he was losing his hearing, but no one knew for certain. In the end, the diagnosticians suspected that his inner ear was injured due to his own body's misguided immune reaction. For some reason, his body had attacked his inner ear as foreign and in need of destruction. At the university speech and hearing clinic, in addition to audiological diagnostic services, Toast received aural rehabilitation, including speechreading, in anticipation of deafness. He was also given behind-the-ear hearing aids.

Eventually Toast lost functional hearing, and his hearing aids were essentially useless. He was diagnosed with bilateral profound sensorineural hearing loss, and when he turned 17, he met all of the requirements for a cochlear implant. Fortunately, he was healthy, with no medical conditions that would prohibit the surgery. Most important, Toast and his family had realistic expectations about its effects and likely benefits. They understood that cochlear implants do not restore normal hearing and that the benefits vary greatly. According to the audiologist, Toast could expect improved sound awareness and, consequently, an improved ability to read lips. Optimally, he might have

Clinical Sidebar 9.4
Rush Limbaugh, the conservative talk show host, and Heather Whitestone McCallum, a former Miss America, have received cochlear implants. Can you name other well-known persons who have had these implants? Do you personally know of such an individual?

improved auditory perception and might be able to comprehend the speech of others even over the telephone. The audiologist suggested a "wait and see" philosophy about the outcome.

Toast met with the cochlear implant team, consisting of an otologist, audiologist, speech-language pathologist, social worker, and Toast's parents. The team discussed several types of cochlear implants and their relative benefits. All cochlear implants include a headset, speech processor, battery source, and a surgically implanted receiver. The audiologist described Toast's candidacy for the procedure and how the processor would be programmed to maximize his auditory perception and speech discrimination. The otologist discussed the outpatient surgery using charts and diagrams. The speech-language pathologist reviewed the speech pathology services Toast would receive. The audiologist and speech-language pathologist explored the follow-up rehabilitative services necessary to maximize the benefits of the cochlear implant.

The surgery began at 8:00 a.m. in the otologist's office, and by 9:30 it was complete. Toast had to wait nearly a month for the *hookup,* in which the audiologist programmed and fit the headset to the processor, a procedure that took about 2 hours. During this important time, the audiologist assessed the ability of the cochlear implant to decipher the acoustic signal into neural impulses. This clinician instructed Toast and his family on how to maintain the system, including changing the batteries and adjusting the controls. About a week after the initial hookup, a second programming session reevaluated the total functioning of the device. A follow-up session occurred several weeks later.

The results of the cochlear implant were better than anticipated. Toast could hear and understand much of the speech of others at normal conversational levels. The improved hearing dramatically improved his speechreading ability as well. The speech sounds produced at the back of a person's mouth are difficult to read, and with the improved hearing provided by the cochlear implant, Toast could either hear or speechread most of what others were saying. The most unexpected and positive aspect of the cochlear implant was that he could now hear his own voice. It had been years since he could clearly hear what he was saying; now, with the implant, he could monitor his pitch and loudness levels. The cochlear implant had returned auditory feedback and continuity to his life. Now in high school halls, even during noisy breaks, he turned to acknowledge friends when they beckoned him: "Yo, Toast."

Case Study 9.5 Social Implications of Deafness and Cochlear Implants

THE ASSOCIATION FOR BETTER COMMUNICATION

You feel honored to be invited to the 3-day, 2-night canoeing and camping trip. You are also pleasantly surprised at the invitation because you are the only hearing person in the group. Canoeing and camping in this northern state promise to be exciting, and

Clinical Sidebar 9.5
In the past, it was not uncommon to see "deaf" individuals soliciting donations in airports, malls, and other public places. They often offered cards with finger-spelling and signs in return for money. Some gave out pencils with quotes or printed signs asking for money. To the ire of the deaf community, many of these persons were charlatans pretending to be deaf. Why did so many in the deaf community respond with outrage? Do you consider deafness a disability? Why or why not?

the fly-fishing is reported to be excellent. You will certainly catch the limit of large mouth bass and trout each day and cook them over an open fire at night. However, as a precaution, your friends decide to purchase freeze-dried snacks, cans of beans, and ready-to-eat meals just in case the fishing is disappointing. You and the group walk through the large shopping mall seeking supplies and provisions, using animated signs, gestures, and facial expression. Many people stop and stare.

In the corner of the mall sits a man begging for money because of deafness, and offering small cards showing finger-spelling and basic signs in return for donations. When your friends see him, they immediately storm toward him and you know an altercation will soon erupt. Your friends are activists in the Association for Better Communication (ABC), and they have little tolerance for deaf beggars.

Just as you feared, a confrontation begins, drawing a crowd of onlookers. Although most of the activists use only sign language, some are capable of speech and they attack the beggar with both. The speech is for the benefit of the growing crowd, and also because the activists believe the beggar may be a con man feigning deafness for money. Soon a security officer arrives to protect the beggar and disperse the crowd. Afterward, the ABC activists and you continue shopping for camping and fishing supplies.

The canoeing and camping adventure begins early Saturday morning, as four canoes and one small rubber raft filled with supplies slide into the picturesque river. You and one of the younger women paddle the third canoe quietly through the winding river. After the group stops for lunch, you and your canoe partner change positions. She is now at the front of the canoe, with you at the back. Soon the river loses its tranquility. As it picks up increasing speed around a bend, you see the rapids. Your canoeing partner is distracted while trying to locate sun block lotion in a back-pack. Suddenly, directly ahead is a large collapsed tree nearly blocking the river. There is only a small area for your canoe to pass, and immediate action is necessary. You shout to your partner to paddle to the left side of the river as quickly as possible. Then, realizing that shouting is not likely to draw her attention, you probe her with your paddle and point to the tree. Just in time, disaster is averted.

That evening, after the group feasts on one small freshly caught trout, and the just-in-case foodstuffs, the discussion turns to cochlear implants. A heated argument quickly develops about the social pros and cons of this new technology that reportly restores partial hearing. Two campers strongly oppose it, arguing that deafness is not a disability but rather a linguistic minority condition. They describe their pride in the deaf community and believe that no surgery should make them something they are not: hearing persons. They also argue that surgeons, audiologists, teachers, and therapists work in their own interests; their professions depend on it. According to the two campers, they should leave "well enough alone." They take pride in their language and culture and are perfectly content with who they are.

Two other campers are equally adamant that deaf persons should be given the opportunity to hear. They note that deafness can be a deterrent to some occupations and professions, and that even with the Americans with Disabilities Act, the freedom and vocational opportunities for people with deafness can be limited. Cochlear implants can be given to very young children, they say, creating learning opportunities previously unavailable. One camper comments on the reality of deafness, using the narrowly averted canoeing disaster as an example. Even though cochlear implants do not restore or create normal hearing, he observes, a person with the device could easily have been warned, reducing the risk of potential drowning.

The trip with your deaf friends has been an exciting wilderness adventure. In the end, you have learned a lot about canoeing and camping, as well as the wisdom of not relying on your fishing prowess as the sole source of food. You also appreciate how deeply some in the deaf community feel about their language and culture, and the challenges the emerging technology of cochlear implants is bringing to their sense of community.

Case Study 9.6 Traumatically Induced Hearing Loss in a 24-Year-Old Man

SEBASTIAN GLASS

Who among us has not done something incredibly stupid and walked away from it unscathed? Darting through traffic outside a crosswalk, cutting off a driver to get onto an exit ramp, skiing the advanced slope without being an expert skier, petting a stray dog, redlining a motorcycle just to see what it can do, and bolting a bicycle though congested traffic are the kinds of things everyone has done at some time without dire consequences. And then there are the kinds of things some of us have done under the influence of alcohol, when the stupidity index is raised. Usually no harm is done, but sometimes intoxication and chance-taking do not mix, and on one Saturday night, Sebastian Glass's luck ran out.

The two couples had been close friends since high school, and clubbing had been a big part of their social lives. Friday and Saturday nights were party nights, and the four longtime friends were hard drinkers. They particularly liked to build a campfire at the deserted army base, tap kegs, and drink into the early morning. On the base was an old two-story wooden geodesic dome, a remnant of army architectural experimentation, and one evening, Sebastian Glass was challenged to climb it. Filled with liquid courage, this fledgling rock climber agreed.

The decrepit building had several footholds, and soon Sebastian was spidering up it. When he reached the top, he stood triumphantly with his hands held high above his head. Then, according to his girlfriend, his footing gave way and he toppled more than two stories, slamming his head onto a concrete pad. Emergency medical technicians brought the unconscious man to the emergency room of a nearby hospital. According

Clinical Sidebar 9.6
Humans can localize sound, that is, know the direction of a sound source, without seeing it. For efficient sound localization, hearing in both ears is necessary. Why? What are the physics of sound localization?

to their report, blood and possibly brain matter were exuding from his right ear at the accident scene. Sebastian spent several weeks in the hospital's acute care section in a coma.

Because of the force of the impact, Sebastian had suffered a severe traumatic brain injury. Weeks later, as he gradually came out of the coma, he was transferred to the hospital's rehabilitation unit, where he underwent extensive neuropsychological and speech-language pathology testing. The test results were suspect, possibly due to Sebastian's traumatically induced hearing loss, and he was then sent to the hospital's audiology section for extensive audiological testing.

Sebastian's fall had nearly torn off his pinna, and there was bleeding and inflammation of his external right ear. The audiologist and otologist administered a battery of tests to the occasionally stuporous man, including an otoscopic examination and pure tones, tympanometry, acoustic reflex, otoacoustic emissions, and brainstem auditory evoked tests. Based on the test results, Sebastian was found to have significant bilateral hearing loss. The ossicular chain of his right ear was disrupted, causing a 55-dB conductive hearing loss. Because of the impact to the skull and the accompanying acceleration and deceleration forces, there was also apparent damage to Sebastian's left cochlea, with corresponding sensorineural hearing loss. A later complication affecting Sebastian's hearing was meningitis, which may have further damaged his auditory processing.

After the testing was completed, the audiologist met with Sebastian's rehabilitation team and his family to discuss the results. He explained the results of the testing and presented charts showing where Sebastian's hearing was damaged. Eventually, Sebastian underwent surgery to repair the ossicular chain in his right ear, and the results were successful. Reconstructive surgery also repaired the damage to his pinna. The audiologist provided amplification for his left ear. At first, this involved a hearing aid donated to the hospital by the family of a deceased patient. Later, Sebastian was given a digital hearing aid. The surgery and amplification helped him to benefit from rehabilitation, and eventually he was discharged to an assisted care facility. After several years, Sebastian was transferred to his parents' home. Today he works in a sheltered environment, sorting and cleaning donated clothing.

SUMMARY

Although considered the second sense after vision, hearing is the primary sense for learning speech and language. Hearing loss and deafness can be serious disabilities, significantly affecting the quality of life. The hearing mechanism converts acoustic energy to mechanical, hydraulic, and electrochemical energy, allowing the person to sense, perceive, and decode speech and environmental sounds. During the past 20 years, audiology technology has improved, allowing all persons to be tested, regardless of their age, level of consciousness, or cooperation, and to learn the status of their hearing mechanism. Technology has brought higher quality amplification to hearing aid wearers, and cochlear implants have opened up a world of better hearing to thousands of persons.

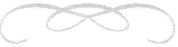

Study and Discussion Questions

1. Draw a sketch of the human ear and identify the major anatomical structures of the external, middle, and inner ears. How are the human ear and its hearing mechanism different from those of other animals, such as cats and dogs?

2. What are the three general types of hearing loss and their typical causes?

3. What is tinnitus? What are some adjectives used to describe it?

4. What hearing tests can be used for newborns, infants, and hard-to-test populations? How might an infant not identified as deaf be misdiagnosed as mentally retarded?

5. What is an air-bone gap, and what is its diagnostic importance?

6. How do hearing aids work? What types of hearing aids exist? Compare the quality of music heard on CD players and satellite radio with that of cassette tapes and older vinyl records. What is the analogy between these devices and the newer and older hearing aid technologies?

7. In middle ear testing, what are compliance, stapedial reflex, and positive and negative air pressure?

8. How do cochlear implants work?

9. What is the technical difference between aural habilitation and aural rehabilitation?

10. Compare and contrast aural habilitation and rehabilitation for children and adults.

11. Provide the arguments for and against the manualist, oralist, and total communication philosophies.

12. Should deafness be considered a disability or should persons who are deaf be viewed as a repressed linguistic minority?

Recommended Reading

Martin, F., & Clark, J. (2003). *Introduction to audiology* (8th ed.). Boston: Allyn & Bacon.
    This comprehensive introductory textbook provides basic information on hearing loss and deafness.

Schow, R., & Nerbonne, M. (Eds.). (2002). *Introduction to audiologic rehabilitation* (4th ed.). Boston: Allyn & Bacon.
    This comprehensive textbook addresses all important aspects of habilitation and re-habilitation for the deaf and hard-of-hearing.

References

Footnotes, the little dogs yapping at the heels of the text

William James

Alvarez, L., & Kolker, A. (1987). *American tongues: A film.* New York: Center for NewAmerican Media.

American Association on Mental Retardation (2002). *Definition of mental retardation.* Retrieved July 8, 2004, from http://www.aamr.org/Policies/fag_mental_retardation.shtml

American Speech-Language-Hearing Association. (2001). *Roles of speech-language pathologists in swallowing and feeding disorders: Position statement.* ASHA Supplement. Rockville, MD: Author.

Aronson, A. E. (1990). *Clinical voice disorders: An interdisciplinary approach* (3rd ed.). New York: Thieme.

Arvedson, J. C., & Brodsky, L. (2002). *Pediatric swallowing and feeding: Assessment and management* (2nd ed.). San Diego, CA: Singular.

Barkley, R. A. (1997). *ADHD and the nature of self-control.* New York: Guilford.

Bass, N. H. (1997). The neurology of swallowing. In M. E. Groher (Ed.), *Dysphagia: Diagnosis and management* (3rd ed., pp. 7–35). Boston: Butterworth-Heinemann.

Bloodstein, O. (1981). *A handbook on stuttering.* Chicago: National Easter Seal Society.

Bloodstein, O. (1995). *A handbook on stuttering* (5th ed.). San Diego, CA: Singular.

Brutten, G. J., & Shoemaker, D. (1967). *The modification of stuttering.* Upper Saddle River, NJ: Prentice Hall.

Byrne, A., Walsh, M., Farrelly, M., & O'Driscoll, K. (1993). Depression following laryngectomy. *British Journal of Psychiatry, 163,* 173–176.

Catts, H. (1996). Defining dyslexia as a developmental language disorder: An expanded view. *Topics in Language Disorders, 16*(2), 14–29.

Cefalu, C. (1999). Appropriate dysphagia evaluation and management of the nursing home patient with dementia. *Annals of Long-Term Care, 7*(12), 447–451.

Chomsky, N. (1980). Human language and other semiotic systems. In T. A. Sebok & J. U. Sebok (Eds.), *Speaking of Apes: A critical anthology of two-way communication with man* (pp. 429–440). New York: Plenum.

Code, C., Hemsley, G., & Herrmann, M. (1999). The emotional impact of aphasia. *Seminars in Speech and Language, 20*(1), 19–31.

Crichton-Smith, I. (2002). Communicating in the real world: Accounts from people who stammer. *Journal of Fluency Disorders, 27*(2002), 333–352.

Culbertson, W., & Tanner, D. (2001a). Clinical comparisons: Phonological processes and their relationship to traditional phoneme norms. *Infant-Toddler Intervention, 11*(1), 15–25.

Culbertson, W., & Tanner, D. (2001b). *Dependency of neuromotor oral maturation on phonological development.* Presented at the 9th Manchester Phonology Meeting, University of Manchester, Manchester, United Kingdom.

Daniels, S., McAdams, C., Brailey, K., & Foundas, A. (1997). Clinical assessment of swallowing and prediction of dysphagia severity. *American Journal of Speech-Language Pathology, 6,* 17–24.

Darley, F. (1982). *Aphasia.* Philadelphia: Saunders.

Darley, F., Aronson, A., & Brown, J. (1975). *Motor speech disorders.* Philadelphia: Saunders.

Davis, G. A. (2000). *Aphasiology: Disorders and clinical practice.* Boston: Allyn & Bacon.

Denning, S. (2000). *The springboard: How storytelling ignites action in knowledge-era organizations.* Boston: Butterworth-Heinemann.

Dirckx, J. H. (2001). *Stedman's concise medical dictionary for the health professions* (4th ed.). Philadelphia: Lippincott Williams & Wilkins.

Duffy, J. (1995). *Motor speech disorders.* St. Louis: Mosby.

Duffy, J. R., & Baumgartner, J. (1997). Psychogenic stuttering in adults with and without neurologic disease. *Journal of Medical Speech-Language Pathology, 5*(2), 75–95.

Eisenson, J. (1984). *Adult aphasia* (2nd ed.). Upper Saddle River, NJ: Prentice Hall.

English, K. (2002). Audiologic rehabilitation services in the school setting. In R. L. Schow & M. A. Nerbonne (Eds.), *Introduction to audiologic rehabilitation* (4th ed., pp. 247–272). Boston: Allyn & Bacon.

Fitzhenry, R. (1993). *The Harper book of quotations* (3rd ed.). New York: HarperPerennial.

Fuller, G. N., & Goodman, J. C. (2001). *Practical review of neuropathology.* Philadelphia: Lippincott Williams & Wilkins.

Ghajar, J. (2000). Traumatic brain injury. *Lancet, 356,* 923–929.

Gillis, R. (1996). *Traumatic brain injury rehabilitation for speech-language pathologists.* Boston: Butterworth-Heinemann.

Gillis, R., & Pierce, J. (1996). Mechanism of traumatic brain injury and the pathophysiologic consequences. In R. Gillis (Ed.), *Traumatic brain injury rehabilitation for speech-language pathologists* (pp. 38–54). Boston: Butterworth-Heinemann.

Gobl, C., & Ni' Chasaide, A. (2002). The role of voice quality in communicating emotion, mood and attitude. *Speech Communication, 40*(1–2), 189–212.

Goldstein, K. (1948). *Language and language disturbances.* New York: Grune & Stratton.

Goldstein, K. (1952). The effects of brain damage on the personality. *Psychiatry, 15,* 245–260.

Guitar, B. (1998). *Stuttering: An integrated approach to its nature and treatment.* Philadelphia: Lippincott Williams & Wilkins.

Hegde, M. N. (2001). *Hedge's pocket guide to treatment in speech-language pathology* (2nd ed.). San Diego, CA: Singular.

Hickey, J. (1997). Craniocerebral injuries: In J. Hickey (Ed.), *The clinical practice of neurological and neurosurgical nursing* (4th ed., pp. 351–394). Philadelphia: Lippincott Williams & Wilkins.

Hirsch, D. (1998). Ask the doctor: Pervasive developmental disorders. *The Exceptional Parent,* Oradell, NJ.

Holmes, A. E. (2002). Cochlear implants and other rehabilitative areas. In R. Schow & M. Nerbonne (Eds.), *Introduction to audiologic rehabilitation* (4th ed., pp. 81–99). Boston: Allyn & Bacon.

Huttlinger, K., & Tanner, D. (1994). The peyote way: Implications for culture care nursing. *Journal of Transcultural Nursing, 5*(2), 5–11.

Johnson, W. (1938). The role of evaluation in stuttering behavior. *Journal of Speech Disorders, 3,* 85–89.

Kagan, S., & Kagan, M. (1998). *Multiple intelligences: The complete MI book.* San Clemente, CA: Kagan Cooperative Learning.

Kent, R. D. (1997). *The speech sciences.* San Diego, CA: Singular.

Klimas, N. (2003). Pediatric audiology: Strategies for working with difficult-to-test children. *Advance, 13*(51).

Kreisler, A., Godefory, O., Delmaire, C., Debachy, B., Leclercq, M., Pruvo, J. P., et al. (2000). The anatomy of aphasia revisited. *Neurology, 54,* 1117–1123.

Kroll, R. M., & DeNil, L. F. (1998). Positron emission tomography studies of stuttering: Their relationship to our theoretical and clinical understanding of the disorder. *Journal of Speech-Language Pathology and Audiology, 22*(4), 261–270.

Ladefoged, P., & Maddieson, I. (1988). *Language, speech and mind: Studies in honour of Victoria Fromkin* (pp. 49–61). London: Routledge.

Laraia, M. (1998). Biological context of psychiatric nursing care. In G. Stuart & M. Laraia (Eds.), *Principles and practice of psychiatric nursing* (6th ed., pp. 82–112). St. Louis: Mosby.

Linn, G. W., & Caruso, A. J. (1998). Perspectives on the effects of stuttering on the formation and maintenance of intimate relationships. *Journal of Rehabilitation, 64*(3), 12–14.

Logemann, J. A. (1998). *Evaluation and treatment of swallowing disorders.* Austin, TX: Pro-Ed.

Mackay, L., Chapman, P., & Morgan, A. (1997). *Maximizing brain injury recovery: Integrating critical care and early rehabilitation.* Gaithersburg, MD: Aspen.

MacNeil, B., Weischselbaum, R., & Pauker, S. (1981). Tradeoffs between quality and quality of life in laryngeal cancer. *New England Journal of Medicine, 305,* 983–987.

Malkmus, D., Booth, B., & Kodimer, C. (1980). *Rehabilitation of the head injured adult: Comprehensive cognitive management.* Downey, CA: Rancho Los Amigos Hospital.

Marquardt, T. P. (2000). Acquired neurogenic language disorders. In R. Gillam, T. Marquardt, & F. Martin (Eds.), *Communication sciences and disorders: From science to clinical practice* (pp. 461–485). San Diego, CA: Singular.

Martin, F. (1997). *Introduction to audiology* (6th ed.). Boston: Allyn & Bacon.

Martin, F., & Clark, J. (2003). *Introduction to audiology* (8th ed.). Boston: Allyn & Bacon.

Moeller, M., Schow, R., & Johnson, D. (2002). Audiologic rehabilitation for children: Assessment and management. In R. Schow and M. Nerbonne (Eds.), *Introduction to audiologic rehabilitation* (4th ed., pp. 277–332). Boston: Allyn & Bacon.

Mueller, H. G., & Carter, A. S. (2002). Hearing aids and assistive devices. In R. Schow & M. Nerbonne (Eds.), *Introduction to audiologic rehabilitation* (4th ed., pp. 31–78). Boston: Allyn & Bacon.

Nelson, J. A. (2000). Audiologic rehabilitation. In R. Gillam, T. Marquardt, & F. Martin (Eds.), *Communication sciences and disorders: From science to clinical practice* (pp. 147–175). San Diego, CA: Singular.

Nicolosi, L., Harryman, E., & Kresheck, J. (2004). *Terminology of communication disorders: Speech-language-hearing* (5th ed.). Philadelphia: Lippincott Williams & Wilkins.

Northern, J. L., & Downs, M. P. (2002). *Hearing in children* (5th ed.). Baltimore: Lippincott Williams & Wilkins.

Owens, R. (1995). *Language disorders: A functional approach to assessment and intervention* (2nd ed.). Boston: Allyn & Bacon.

Owens, R. (2001). *Language development: An introduction* (5th ed.). Boston: Allyn & Bacon.

Owens, R., Metz, D., & Haas, A. (2000). *Introduction to communication disorders.* Boston: Allyn & Bacon.

Ozonoff, S., Dawson, G., & McPartland, J. (2002). *A parent's guide to Asperger syndrome and high-functioning autism: How to meet the challenges and help your child thrive.* New York: Guilford.

Perlman, A. L., & Christensen, J. (1997). Topography and functional anatomy of the swallowing structures. In A. L. Perlman & K. S. Schulze-Delrieu (Eds.), *Deglutition and its disorders: Anatomy, physiology, clinical diagnosis, and management* (pp. 15–42). San Diego, CA: Singular.

Petit, J. M. (2001). *Primary neurologic care.* St. Louis: Mosby.

Pichora-Fuller, K., & Schow, R. (2002). Audiologic rehabilitation for adults and elderly adults: Assessment and management. In R. L. Schow & M. A. Nerbonne (Eds.), *Introduction to audiologic rehabilitation* (4th ed., pp. 335–397). Boston: Allyn & Bacon.

Plante, E., & Beeson, P. (2004). *Communication and communication disorders: A clinical introduction* (2nd ed.). Boston: Allyn & Bacon.

Ramig, L. O., & Verdolini, K. (1998). Treatment efficacy: Voice disorders. *Journal of Speech, Language, and Hearing Research, 41,* S101–S116.

Restak, R. (1984). *The brain.* Toronto: Bantam Books.

Rollin, W. J. *Counseling individuals with communication disorders: Psychodynamics and family aspects* (2nd ed.). Boston: Butterworth-Heinemann.

Schmidt, C., Andrews, M. L., & McCutcheon, J. W. (1998). An acoustical and perceptual analysis of the vocal behavior of classroom teachers. *Journal of Voice, 12*(4), 434–443.

Schow, R., & Nerbonne, M. (Eds.). (2002). Introduction to audiologic rehabilitation. Boston: Allyn & Bacon.

Smeltzer, D., Nasrallah, H., & Miller, S. (1994). Psychotic disorders. In J. Silver, S. Yudofsky, & R. Hales (Eds.), *Neuropsychiatry of traumatic brain injury* (pp. 251–283). Washington, DC: American Psychiatric Press.

Smith, E., Kirchner, L. H., Taylor, M., Hoffman, H., & Lemke, J. H. (1998). Voice problems among teachers: Differences by gender and teacher characteristics. *Journal of Voice, 12*(3), 328–334.

Spahr, F., & Malone, R. (1998). The profession of speech-language pathology and audiology. In G. Shames, E. Wiig, & W. Secord (Eds.), *Human communication disorders: An introduction* (5th ed., pp. 1–26). Boston: Allyn & Bacon.

Sparks, R., Helm, N., & Albert, N. (1974). Aphasia rehabilitation resulting from melodic intonation therapy. *Cortex, 10,* 303–316.

Stemple, J. C. (1984). *Clinical voice pathology: Theory and management.* Columbus, OH: Merrill.

Stone, A. C., Silliman, E. R., Ehren, B. J., & Apel, K. (Eds.). (2004). *Handbook of language and literacy: Development and disorders.* New York: Guilford.

Tanner, D. (1980). Loss and grief: Implications for the speech-language pathologist and audiologist. *ASHA, 22,* 916–928.

Tanner, D. (1990a). *Muscular relaxation training program for voice disorders.* Oceanside, CA: Academic Communication Associates.

Tanner, D. (1990b). *Assessment of stuttering behaviors.* Oceanside, CA: Academic Communication Associates.

Tanner, D. (1991). *Relaxation training for stutterers.* Oceanside, CA: Academic Communication Associates.

Tanner, D. (1994). *Pragmatic stuttering intervention for children* (2nd ed.). Oceanside, CA: Academic Communication Associates.

Tanner, D. (1999a). *The family guide to surviving stroke and communication disorders.* Austin: Pro-Ed.

Tanner, D. (1999b). *Understand stuttering: A guide for parents.* Oceanside, CA: Academic Communication Associates.

Tanner, D. (2003a). *The psychology of neurogenic communication disorders: A primer for health care professionals.* Boston: Allyn & Bacon.

Tanner, D. (2003b). *The forensic aspects of communication sciences and disorders.* Tucson, AZ: Lawyers and Judges.

Tanner, D. (2003c). *Exploring communication disorders: A 21st century introduction through literature and media.* Boston: Allyn & Bacon.

Tanner, D. (2003d). Eclectic perspectives on the psychology of aphasia. *Journal of Allied Health, 32,* 256–260.

Tanner, D., Belliveau, W., & Siebert, G. (1995). *Pragmatic stuttering intervention for adolescents and adults.* Oceanside, CA: Academic Communication Associates.

Tanner, D., & Culbertson, W. (1999a). *Quick assessment for dysphagia.* Oceanside, CA: Academic Communication Associates.

Tanner, D., & Culbertson, W. (1999b). *Quick assessment for apraxia of speech.* Oceanside, CA: Academic Communication Associates.

Tanner, D., Culbertson, W., & Secord, W. (1997). *Developmental articulation and phonology profile.* Oceanside, CA: Academic Communication Associates.

Tanner, D., & Gerstenberger, D. (1996). Clinical forum 9: The grief model in aphasia. In C. Code (Ed.), *Forums in clinical aphasiology* (pp. 313–318). London: Whurr.

Tanner, D., & Guzzino, A. (2002, April). *Westlaw search of litigation areas in communication sciences and disorders.* Paper presented at the 2001–2002 Honors Day Program, Northern Arizona University, Flagstaff, AZ.

Tanner, D., & Lafferty, H. (2001). Singing about stuttering. *ASHA Leader, 6*(9), 31.

Tanner, D., Lamb, W., & Secord, W. (1997). *The cognitive, linguistic, and social-communicative scales* (2nd ed.). Oceanside, CA: Academic Communication Associates.

Tanner, D., & Tanner, M. (2004). *The forensic aspects of speech patterns: Voice prints, speaker profiling, lie and intoxication detection.* Tucson, AZ: Lawyers and Judges.

Tanner, D., Weems, L., Nye, C., & Lamb, W. (1988, November). *Direct and indirect correlations of preschool language assessment.* Paper presented at the annual convention of the American Speech-Language-Hearing Association, Boston.

Teasdale, G., & Jennett, B. (1974). Assessment of coma and impaired consciousness: A practical guide. *Lancet, 13,* 81–84.

Terrace, H. S., Petitto, L. A., Sanders, R. J., & Bever, T. B. (1979). Can an ape create a sentence? *Science, 206,* 891–902.

Tetnowski, J. A. (2003). Foreword. In D. Tanner, *The psychology of neurogenic communication disorders: A primer for health care professionals* (pp. ix–xi). Boston: Allyn & Bacon.

Tharpe, A. M. (2004). Disorders of hearing in children. In E. Plante & P. Beeson (Eds.), *Communication and communication disorders: A clinical introduction (*2nd ed., pp. 253–285). Boston: Allyn & Bacon.

Tosi, O., Tanner, D., & Supal, C. (1976). *Acoustic and intelligibility characteristics of Parkinsonian dysarthria.* Paper presented at the International Congress of Logopedia, Phoniatria and Audiologia, Vallodolid, Spain.

U.S. Department of Education. (1997). *To assure the free appropriate public education of all Americans: Nineteenth annual report to Congress on the implementation of the Individuals with Disabilities Education Act.* Publication No. 1997-616-188/90444. Washington, DC: U.S. Government Printing Office.

Van Riper, C. (1973). *The treatment of stuttering.* Upper Saddle River, NJ: Prentice Hall.

Van Riper, C. (1992). *The nature of stuttering* (2nd ed.). Upper Saddle River, NJ: Prentice Hall. (Reissued by Waveland Press, Prospect Heights, IL.)

Waldowski, K., & Wilkes, B. (2003). Tricks of the trade: Articulation therapy for children with hearing loss. *Advance, 13*(14), 6.

Wise, R. J. S., Greene, J., Büchel, C., & Scott, S. K. (1999). Brain regions involved in articulation. *Lancet, 353,* 1057–1061.

Westby, C. E. (1998). Communicative refinement in school age and adolescence. In W. O. Haynes & B. B. Shulman (Eds.), *Communication development: Foundations, processes, and clinical applications* (pp. 311–360). Baltimore: Lippincott Williams & Wilkins.

Wiig, E. (2004a). Professional correspondence. Manuscript review.

Wiig, E., & Secord, W. (1998). Language disabilities and school-age children and youth. In G. Shames, E. Wiig, & W. Secord (Eds.), *Human communication disorders: An introduction* (5th ed., pp. 185–226). Boston: Allyn & Bacon.

Wiig, K. M. (2004b). *People-focused knowledge management.* Burlington, MA: Elsevier/Butterworth-Heinemann.

Williams, A. C., Sandy, J. R., Thomas, S., Sell, D., & Sterne, J. A. C. (1999). Influence of surgeon's experience on speech outcome in cleft lip and palate. *Lancet, 354,* 1697–1698.

Wise, R. J. S., Greene, J., Büchel, C., & Scott, S. K. (1999). Brain regions involved in articulation. *Lancet, 353,* 1057–1061.

Wolfram, W. (1986). Language variation in the United States. In O. L. Taylor (Ed.), *Nature of communication disorders in culturally and linguistically diverse populations* (pp. 73–115). San Diego, CA: College Hill.

Yellin, W., Culbertson, W., Tanner, D., & Adams, T. (2000a, March). *Newborn hearing screening in a well baby nursery.* Paper presented to the annual convention of the American Academy of Audiology, Chicago.

Yellin, M., Culbertson, W., Tanner, D., & Adams, T. (2000b). Gender differences in transient evoked otoacoustic emissions (TEOAEs) of newborns. *Infant-Toddler Intervention, 10*(3), 177–200.

Ylvisaker, M. (1998). Traumatic brain injury in children and adolescents: Introduction. In M. Ylvisaker (Ed.), *Traumatic brain injury rehabilitation* (2nd ed., pp. 1–10). Boston: Butterworth-Heinemann.

Ylvisaker, M., Szekeres, S. F., & Feeney, T. (2001). Communication disorders associated with traumatic brain injury. In R. Chapey (Ed.), *Language intervention strategies in aphasia and related neurogenic communication disorders* (4th ed., pp. 745–808). Philadelphia: Lippincott Williams & Wilkins.

Zemlin, W. (1998). *Speech and hearing science* (4th ed.). Boston: Allyn & Bacon.

Zwirner P., Murry, T., & Woodson, G. (1991). Phonatory function of neurologically impaired patients. *Journal of Communication Disorders, 24,* 287–300.

Index

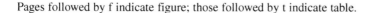

Pages followed by f indicate figure; those followed by t indicate table.